TAKING CHARGE

TAKING CHARGE

Nursing, Suffrage, and
Feminism in America,
1873–1920

Sandra Beth Lewenson

~

NLN Press • New York
Pub. No. 14-6843

ISBN 0-88737-684-3

The views expressed in this book reflect those of the author and do not necessarily reflect the official views of the National League for Nursing.

This book was set in Bembo by Publications Development Company, Crockett, Texas. The designer was Allan Graubard. The printer was BookCrafters. The cover was designed by Lauren Stevens.

Printed in the United States of America.

This book is dedicated to Richard for his scholarly criticism, unfailing patience, and restoring humor, and to Jennifer and Nicole for their support and encouragement.

Contents

Contents

Preface

The nurse question is the woman question pure and simple.

A Character Sketch by an Intimate of
Ethel Gordon Fenwick, 1901.[1]

*. . . if ever a profession had to contend with misunderstanding, mis-
representation, antagonism, and exploitation, it's nursing.*

Sara Parsons, 1917[2]

SINCE 1873 AND the rise of the modern nursing movement, nurses took
charge of their personal and professional lives—a struggle that continues
today. In asserting their independence, many nurses supported the
woman suffrage movement and fulfilled the mission of the social feminists of the late nineteenth and early twentieth century. *Taking Charge:
Nursing, Suffrage, and Feminism in America 1873–1920* describes the
events leading to the professional growth of the trained nurse who replaced the "natural born nurse" following the opening of nurse-training
schools in 1873. Previously, any woman could be called a nurse; in the
home she may have been a family's "spinster" relative, in the hospital she
may have been someone notorious as a slovenly drunk. The changing
roles of women and the subsequent changes in family life as American
society moved from an agrarian to industrial nation affected the health
of American cities and their residents. The devastating effects of over-
crowding, poverty, and questionable sanitary practices provided the impetus for several Progressive Era reform movements in which the newly
trained nurse found opportunity for valuable service to society.

In 1893, twenty years after the opening of the first Nightingale-
influenced nurse training schools in America, the first nursing

organizations were formed. These organizations focused on essential requirements of the emerging profession for quality education, legal status for professionally trained nurses, and improved working conditions. Through the collective action of nursing organizations, nurses joined other women's groups in their efforts to improve the social, political, and economic conditions of women. In keeping with the spirit of the late nineteenth and early twentieth century woman movement, professional nursing organizations supported the woman suffrage movement.

Taking Charge does not intend to be a complete history of nursing; instead it scrutinizes one aspect that has often been neglected or inaccurately assessed. The book examines the way women established the nursing profession outside of the acceptable but separate sphere of domesticity. Nursing pioneers constantly struggled with paternalistic ideology that impinged on their freedom to control education and practice for the nursing profession and promoted the concept that any woman could be a nurse, in spite of the evidence indicating the importance of education in reducing mortality and morbidity rates. Pioneer nursing leaders had to form powerful coalitions among themselves in order to overcome opponents of nursing's professional activities. Professional nursing organizations became political strongholds in which nurses collectively combated the ignorance surrounding nursing care. They raised the standards of nursing practice, nursing education, and nursing administration. As they sought control of their own professional and personal destinies, they learned that they needed woman suffrage to transform their ideas into reality. Many nurses reasoned that their goal of state registration to protect the public from untrained nurses would never be achieved without the vote. Consequently, by 1912, the two oldest national nursing organizations officially supported woman suffrage.

The history of this period reveals the stirring and admirable accomplishments of the nursing leaders of the late nineteenth and early twentieth century. Nurses thoughtfully considered and addressed the social problems that affected health care and showed great concern for improving both the care of the sick and the care of the well. Through the leadership of the professional nursing organizations between 1893 and 1910, nurses demonstrated a constant interest in their own professional growth; later, between 1911 and 1920, they expanded their focus to include more global concerns affecting women's rights.

Research into the relationship between nursing, suffrage, and feminism has revealed the unacknowledged earlier contributions of nursing to the suffrage movement and the larger woman movement, contributions which have remained unnoticed by nurses, women, and society at large. This omission from women's studies, United States women's history, and from nursing historiographies constitutes tacit support of the generally tarnished and devalued image of the nursing profession that has persisted through the years. Although I assumed that most people knew that Lillian Wald (1867–1940) founded the Henry Street Settlement, supported woman suffrage, and advocated world peace, I was unaware that many did not know that Wald was a nurse. In my daughter's high school history text, *The National Experience: A History of the United States,* Wald is referred to as a social reformer, with no mention of her professional work as a nurse.[3] The only reference to nursing in this popular text describes this profession as part of a "feminine ghetto," thus relegating its college-educated and trained practitioners to the low status of other women-dominated professions. This cavalier stereotyping of the profession of nursing denies its potential as an exciting career prospect for contemporary high school students of both genders.

I hope that *Taking Charge* will inform the reader of the significance of nursing's rich history of practice, education, and professionalization of women's work and promote inclusion of this history into the general curriculum of schools, colleges, and universities. Health care professionals, in particular, need to understand the history of nursing and to acknowledge the political and economic tensions that persist in the late twentieth century as a result of the paternalism that permeates the health care model we know today.

Because the interpretation of history is often clouded by contemporary perceptions, historiography requires the removal and refocusing of a contemporary lens in order to present and interpret an unbiased view of the past. *Taking Charge* examines the activities of the four national nursing organizations that formed between 1893 and 1912 through the records of their proceedings and through articles and essays by trained nurses published in nursing journals between 1893 and 1920. The sources reveal that nurses actively engaged in the promotion of woman's rights and sought changes predicated on their sense of collectivity, their female consciousness, and their outright feminism.[4]

Nurses' support of women's issues directly related to their attainment of professional nursing goals. Trained nurses worked to support themselves, and in doing so, embodied the ideological framework of the woman movement which emphasized women's need for financial independence, higher education, and personal autonomy. The position that nurses and nursing leaders took in regard to woman's rights focused on what was useful and practical to the developing profession as a whole. The pioneering generation of nurses hoped that woman suffrage would translate into professional autonomy for nurses.

The nursing profession and its role in society has been associated inextricably with the traditional role of women. In 1973, nurse and feminist Wilma Scott Heide (1921–1985) wrote of the ease with which the term "nurse" was substituted for the term "woman" when discussing so-called feminine traits. Women and nurses shared stereotypical qualities such as caring, nurturing, compassion, tenderness, submissiveness, passivity, subjectiveness, and emotionalism.[5] While some of these traits enhance the performance of the professional role of nurses, others serve to inhibit the autonomy of nursing professionals. How could one be caring and submissive and still advocate the rights of nurses or patients in the health care system? Historian Susan Reverby sums up this dilemma, arguing that nurses were required to care "in a society that refuses to value caring."[6]

Paradoxically, nursing has been described as a metaphor for the ". . . struggle of women for equality."[7] Contemporary nursing scholarship has begun to reflect nursing's identification with women's issues in the past twenty years, as well as in the woman movement of the early twentieth century.[8] The collective efforts through which women moved into the public sphere and advocated social reform began in 1848 and continued to be referred to as the "woman movement" at the beginning of this century. A number of different woman's groups fell under their umbrella, and the term "woman movement" has been used interchangeably with the term "feminism."[9] Feminism has been defined by contemporary nursing authors as "a world view that values women and that confronts systematic injustices based on gender."[10] In *Taking Charge,* the efforts to value women and their contributions in all areas of life define the term "feminism;" the term "feminist movement" refers to the women's movement in the 1960s and 1970s, and "woman movement" indicates the earlier movement in American history beginning with the meeting at Seneca Falls in 1848 until the passage of the Nineteenth Amendment in 1920. The concept of "practical feminism" will be applied to the activities of professional nursing that pursued an informed status for women in the profession at the end of the nineteenth and the beginning of the twentieth century.

Despite the links between the profession of nursing and the women's movement, nursing scholarship often depicts a strained relationship between these two efforts. Nursing and nurses often seemed to embody the very characteristics and problems that feminists challenged. As a result of this tension, the goal of feminism to broaden women's opportunities has been assumed to obscure the profession of nursing and to exclude its empowerment of women through its dynamic career opportunities. At times, feminist leadership has failed to look beyond the perceived, inaccurate sexist stereotype of nurses, or even acknowledge the full potential of the nursing profession.[11]

Feminists in the 1960s and 1970s expressed their opposition to male-defined systems and ideologies that systematically oppress women. A breach developed between feminists and nurses because of some feminists' perception of nursing as the embodiment of woman's submissive role and nursing's admission in the professional nursing literature of its having become male-defined, male-dominated, and therefore systematically oppressed. Friction between the nursing profession and the feminist movement evolved because feminists opposed male-defined systems and nursing has been perceived as the creature of a totally male-defined system.[12] The origins of feminism and nursing in United States women's history, studied together, reveal the true nature of the exchange and interaction between these two movements of the late nineteenth and early twentieth century.

Chapter One, the introduction "From Separate to Active Spheres," offers an inclusive examination of women's history and nursing's history between 1850 to 1893. This chapter explains the impact of the changing roles of women and men during this era on women's education, nursing education, and American health care as it describes the shared history of the woman movement, the woman suffrage movement, and the modern nursing movement. Moreover, this chapter introduces the major historical figures who contributed to women's education, nursing education, and women's advance from the separate, domestic sphere to the collective, active sphere.

Professional nursing eschewed the limitations of the "born" nurse ideology and pursued emancipation as a self-determined group through the formation of nursing organizations beginning in 1893. Chapter Two, "Emancipation Through Organization," presents an historical account of the formation of four national nursing organizations between 1893 and 1920. The first of these organizations, the American Society of Superintendents of Training Schools for Nurses (hereafter the Superintendents' Society), was established in 1893, renamed the National League of Nursing Education (NLNE) in 1912, and became the National League for Nursing (NLN) in 1952. Three years later, the Nurses' Associated Alumnae of the United States and Canada (hereafter the Associated Alumnae), formed in 1896 and was renamed the American Nurses' Association (ANA) in 1911. The National Association of Colored Graduate Nurses (NACGN), established in 1908, existed until 1952 when it affiliated with the American Nurses' Association. Finally, the National Organization for Public Health Nursing (NOPHN), founded in 1912, joined the National League for Nurses in 1952. This second chapter describes the nursing leaders whose ideas shaped American nursing and influenced their participation as individuals and within professional organizations in the woman movement. Since these four national organizations illustrate the profession's efforts to control the advancement of nursing during the late nineteenth and early twentieth century, the chapter summarizes the history of each organization. In addition, this chapter describes the significant role the American Federation of Nurses, an affiliation established between the Superintendents' Society and the Associated Alumnae, played in representing American nurses to other national and international women's organizations. The description of each organization reveals nursing's collective response to the woman movement.

During "The Formative Years: Nursing and Suffrage, 1893–1910," the focus of Chapter Three, the developing profession addressed specific issues of professional autonomy and self-determination within nursing while the woman movement addressed the inclusive goal of personal advancement of women in society. Key issues such as education, recruitment of new nurses, shorter work hours, and pay equity confronted the nursing profession, while women's organizations faced similar concerns about women's education, political franchise, and work opportunities. Women's rights activists found allies among their nursing counterparts because their interests in social, political, and economic concerns often overlapped. Finding that the resolution of the problems addressed by both nursing and women's organizations could only be achieved through the equal rights of women, nurses advocated suffrage for women. However, nursing's formative years of professional development required that priority be given to establishing precedents, policies, and procedures within the new profession; therefore, its outward support of suffrage did not peak during that period. Nevertheless, the gradual support for woman's rights by nursing's professional organizations originated during the formative years. Between 1893 and 1911, nurses struggled for professional autonomy and found that only through political freedom could they move closer to emancipation from male domination and control of nursing education and practice.

Chapter Four, "The Expanding Years: Nursing Supports Suffrage, 1911–1920," charts the historical context of nurses' formal vote in support of woman suffrage through their professional organizations. By 1912, American nursing had sent a delegation to participate in the passage of an international woman suffrage resolution sponsored by the International Council of Nurses meeting in Cologne, Germany. The nursing profession had moved from a narrow focus on professional development toward a far wider and more active role in the social reforms of the Progressive Era. The exercise of delegate franchise within their nursing organizations moved nurses to demand the same empowerment and equal political participation within the broader society. To this end, nursing's alliances with a variety of women's groups interested in social reforms flourished.

Chapter Five, "Taking Charge," expands on the connections between organized professional nursing and the woman movement and explains the impact of those relationships on contemporary nursing, women, and American health care. The chronic omission of nursing from contemporary historiographies of nineteenth and twentieth century women's history and the continued prejudice towards the caring role of the nurse in society is discussed in this final chapter. I have coined a new term, "nursism," to bridge the semantic gap that stems from an historic disdain of nursing as a woman's profession. Historically, there has existed a condescending assumption that the subordination of the nurse to the physician in the male-dominated medical system has resulted not from the general oppression of women by a patriarchal society, but from collusion by the profession of nursing.[13] Therefore, the term nursism attempts to point to and challenge the prejudice that the profession has experienced and reacted to over time. The term represents the determined defiance of nurses of these efforts to demean them or define them as lesser partners in patient care. Nursism serves to describe this proud movement of people in nursing who have continued to struggle to develop and establish their profession as necessary, respected, specialized, and autonomous.

During the 1990s and into the twenty-first century, we see the increased awareness of the need for an improved, accessible, and affordable health care system in America. Nursing can contribute important services within a holistic health care system that learns to value both the caring and curative roles of different health care professionals within diverse communities. Identifying nursism in history and its role in the history of nursing creates an understanding of the constraints in nursing today and facilitates the search for new paradigms in which to move society toward a more humanistic health care system in the next century.

NOTES

1. A Character Sketch by an Intimate, "Foreign Delegates and Organizations," Ethel Gordon Fenwick, *AJN*, 1 no. 12 (September, 1901): 865. Fenwick was the founder and first president of the International Council of Nurses and the honorary president of the Congress of Nurses at Buffalo, 1901.

2. Sara Parsons, "Address," *Proceedings of the Twenty-third Annual Convention of the NLNE* (Baltimore: Williams and Wilkins, 1917), 56.

3. John M. Blum, William S. McFeely, Edmund S. Morgan, Arthur Schlesinger, Jr., Kenneth M. Stampp, and C. Vann Woodward, *The National Experience: A History of the United States* 6th ed. (San Diego: Harcourt Brace Jovanovich, 1985), 484, 902.

4. Nancy E. Cott, "What's in a Name? The Limits of 'Social Feminism'; or, Expanding the Vocabulary of Women's History," *Journal of American History* 76 (December, 1989): 809–829 to give an explanation; William

O'Neil, *Everyone was Brave: The Rise and Fall of Feminism in America* (Chicago, Quadrangle Books, 1960), ix–x, defines the terms feminist, social feminist, and woman movement.

5. George L. Choon and Suzanne M. Skevington, "How Do Women and Men in Nursing Perceive Each Other?" In *Understanding Nurses,* ed. Suzanne M. Skevington (New York: Wiley & Sons, 1984), 101–111; Janet Muff, ed., *Socialization, Sexism, and Stereotyping: Women's Issues in Nursing* (St. Louis: Mosby, 1982); Wilma Scott Heide "Nursing and Women's Liberation a Parallel," *The American Journal of Nursing,* 73 no. 5 (1973): 824–827. Wilma Scott Heide was president of the National Organization of Women between 1970 and 1974 and author of *Feminism for the Health of It* (Buffalo, NY: Margaretdaughters, 1985).

6. Susan Reverby, *Ordered To Care: The Dilemma of American Nursing, 1850–1945* (Cambridge: Cambridge University Press, 1987), 1.

7. Donna Diers, "To Profess—To Be A Professional," *The Journal of the New York State Nurses Association,* 15 no. 4 (December, 1984): 23

8. Margaret Allen, "Women, Nursing and Feminism: An Interview with Alice J. Baumgart, RN, PhD," *The Canadian Nurse,* 81 no. 1 (January, 1985): 20–22; Linda Andrist, "A Feminist Framework for Graduate Education in Women's Health," *Journal of Nursing Education,* 27 no. 2 (February, 1988): 66–70; Heide, "Nursing and Women's Liberation a Parallel, 824–827; Wilma Scott Heide, *Feminism for the Health of It* (Buffalo, NY: Margaretdaughters, 1985); Angela B. McBride, "A Married Feminist," *The American Journal of Nursing,* 76 no. 5 (May, 1976): 754–757; Dorothy Starr, "Poor Baby: The Nurse and Feminism," *The Canadian Nurse,* 70 no. 3 (March, 1974): 20–23; Susan Talbott and Connie Vance, "Involving Nursing in a Feminist Group—Now," *Nursing Outlook,* 29 no. 10 (October, 1981): 592–595.

9. Nancy F. Cott, *The Grounding of Modern Feminism* (New Haven: Yale University Press, 1987), 3, 12–20; O'Neil, *Everyone Was Brave,* ix–x, for a discussion of the development of the term "feminism."

10. Peggy L. Chinn and Charlene Eldrige Wheeler, "Feminism and Nursing," *Nursing Outlook,* 33 no. 2 (March/April, 1985): 74.

11. Allen, "Women, Nursing and Feminism," 20–22; Ellen Baer, "American Nursing: 100 Years of Conflicting Ideas and Ideals," *The Journal of the New York State Nurses Association,* 23 no. 3 (September, 1992): 19. Baer expresses her disappointment that the late twentieth century "mainstream feminist movement has not taken up the cause of women doing traditional female work." Ellen Baer, "The Feminist Disdain for Nursing," *New York Times,* 23 February, 1991, 25; Vern Bullough and

Bonnie Bullough, *History, Trends, and Politics of Nursing* (Norwalk, CT: Appleton-Century-Crofts, 1984); L. Fitzpatrick, "Nursing," *Signs*, 2:4 (1977): 818–834; and Connie Vance, Susan Talbott, Angela McBride, and D. Mason, "Coming of Age: The Women's Movement and Nursing," in *Political Action Handbook for Nurses*, eds. Diana Mason and Susan Talbott (Menlo Park, CA: Addison Wesley, 1985), 23–37.

12. Jo Ann Ashley, "Nurses in American History, Nursing and Early Feminism," *AJN*, 75 no. 9 (September, 1975); 1465–1467; Jo Ann Ashley, *Hospitals, Paternalism, and the Role of the Nurse* (New York: Teachers College Press, 1976), 123–134; Bullough and Bullough, *History, Trends, and Politics of Nursing*; Chinn and Wheeler, "Feminism and Nursing," 74–77; Heide, Nursing and Women's Liberation," 824–827; Anselm Strauss, "The Structure and Ideology of American Nursing: An Interpretation," in *Nursing Profession: Five Sociological Essays*, ed. Fred Davis (New York: John Wiley and Sons, 1966), 60–108, 87. Strauss notes that nursing formed around "virtuous feminine themes" and were not idealized as "political (equal rights) reformers."

13. Ashley, *Hospitals*, 75–93; Muff, *Socialization, Sexism, and Stereotyping*, 157–168, 203–209, 210–233, 255–272; Phillip Kalisch and Beatrice Kalisch, *The Advance of American Nursing*, 2nd ed. (Boston: Little, Brown & Company, 1986), 216–218, are among the many readings related to nursing's subordinate role in the health care system. A discussion of nursism appears in Sandra Lewenson, *The Relationship Among the Four Professional Nursing Organizations and Woman Suffrage: 1893–1920*, Ed.D. diss., Teachers College, Columbia University, 1989 (Ann Arbor, MI, University Microfilms International, order number 9002561), 179–181, and in Sandra Lewenson, "The Woman's Nursing and Suffrage Movement, 1893–1920," in *Florence Nightingale and Her Era: A Collection of New Scholarship*, eds. Vern Bullough, Bonnie Bullough, and Marietta Stanton (New York: Garland Publishing Company, 1990), 131–132.

Acknowledgments

My attempt to uncover nursing's vital commitment to America's woman movement received a great deal of attention and support from many people. I would like to acknowledge Professors Mae Pepper and Carolyn Lansberry at Mercy College, who fostered my professional creativity through their mentoring and guidance. Patricia Moccia, chief executive officer of the National League for Nursing and my former advisor at Teachers College, Columbia University, explored with me the feminist nature of the early pioneers in nursing and their contributions to the profession. Professor Elaine LaMonica chaired my dissertation committee at Teachers College and supported my independence and expression of ideas. The dissertation committee members, Professors Betty Tucker, Betty Mahoney, and Douglas Sloan worked together, providing me with ample support for my work. My colleagues at Teachers College, Sharon Hudacek, Donna Rinaldi Carpenter, Kathy Scoble, and Marie Mosley, loved the idea of "nursism" from the start and allowed me to explore this concept with them and their students.

My work led me to several libraries and archives and I am indebted to their wonderful staff for assisting me in this work. I especially want to thank archivist Peter Ment and Bette Weneck at Special Collections, Milbank Memorial Library, Teachers College; Adele Lerner at the New York-Cornell Medical Center Archives; Fred Pattison at the American Journal of Nursing Company; Arian Ravanbaksh at Johns Hopkins; Thomas Rosenbaum and Melissa Smith at Rockefeller Archives in Pocantico Hills, New York; Peter Hirtle and Jan Lazarus at the National Library of Medicine; Jack Termine at the State University of New York, Health Science Center at Brooklyn; and Carla Castillo at the Center for the Study of the History of Nursing at University of Pennsylvania, the Schomburg Center for Research in Black Culture in New York, and the Mugar Library in Boston.

Acknowledgments

Throughout the writing of this book, I sought the expertise of other nurse historians and the members of the American Association of the History of Nursing. I am grateful to Nettie Birnbach, Joan Lynaugh, Ellen Baer, and Vern L. Bullough, all of whom freely shared their ideas and thoughts on this project.

My colleagues at State University of New York (SUNY), Health Science Center at Brooklyn, College of Nursing, especially Sandee Fielo, Minerva Guttman, and Daisy-Cruz Richman, supported my enthusiasm for this subject. Nursing students Stephlyn Murray, Rachael Niland, Nadine Louissant, Hyacinth Simmons, Celeste Pate LeFlore, Velma Purcell, Jacqueline Johnson, Konah Gomez, Sandra Hibbert, Morrine Day, and Carol Hanson Beckles were first to enroll in the nursing history elective and enthusiastically discussed the importance of such a course in their professional lives.

I especially want to thank Angela Howard Zophy who has supported this project throughout the various stages and recognized its importance to women's history in America. I also want to thank Merri Scheibe for her careful editing. Further acknowledgment is given to the Zeta Omega Westchester Rockland Chapter at Large, Sigma Theta Tau International Honor Society, which funded a portion of this project.

Among my family and friends I wish to acknowledge for providing endless discussions regarding women's work, women's roles, and nursing are Michelle Kalina, Michael Kalina, Henri Nibur, Pearl Nibur Chandler, Jim Chandler, Billy Nibur, Cindy Nibur, Heather Nibur, Ross Nibur, Barbara Nibur, Joanna Novello, Jean Porges, Leslie Wexler, Sharon Panessa, Joy Jones, Nora Galland, Al Galland, Diana Zimmerman, Sol Zimmerman, Joyce Beldengreen, Gilbert Beldengreen, and Linda Berman. I would like to acknowledge all those friends and colleagues I have not named but who helped me during the many years of writing this book.

Finally, I would like to thank the support I have received for this book since it was completed. I am honored by the American Association of the History of Nursing, for awarding this work the coveted Lavinia L. Dock Award for Historical Scholarship and Research in Nursing. I especially want to thank Allan Graubard, Director of NLN Press, who recognized the importance of this work for present and future researchers and for bringing it to this edition.

List of Abbreviations

AJN	*The American Journal of Nursing*
ANHNC	The Adelaide Nutting Historical Nursing Collection located in the Milbank Memorial Library
Associated Alumnae	Nurses' Associated Alumnae of the United States and Canada
ANA	American Nurses Association
ASSTSN	American Society of Superintendents of Training Schools for Nurses
HMD–NLM	History of Medicine Division, National Library of Medicine, Bethesda, MD
ICN	International Council of Nurses
ICW	International Council of Women
MML	The Milbank Memorial Library, Special Collections, Teachers College, Columbia University, New York
MML–NA	Mugar Memorial Library, Nursing Archives American Nurses Association, Board of Directors Minutes: 1897–1949 (Records of Associated Alumnae of U.S. and Canada, 1897–1912), N87, Boston University, Boston
NACGN	National Association of Colored Graduate Nurses
NACGNR	National Association of Colored Graduate Nurses Records (1908–1951)
NAW	*Notable American Women*

List of Abbreviations

NCW	National Council of Women
NLN	National League for Nursing
NLNE	National League of Nursing Education
NOPHN	National Organization for Public Health Nursing
NYH-CMC	Medical Archives, New York-Hospital-Cornell Medical Center, New York
RAC	Rockefeller Archive Center, Pocantico, New York
RG	Record Group
Schomburg	Schomburg Center for Research in Black Culture, Rare Books, Manuscripts, and Archives Section, New York Public Library, New York
Superintendents' Society	American Society of Superintendents of Training Schools for Nurses
TC-CU	Teachers College, Columbia University, New York
TN	Trained Nurse

Glossary

TERMS USED IN the emerging profession of nursing during the late nineteenth and early twentieth century.

TERM	DEFINITION
probationer	Student during the first few months of nurse training.
private duty nurse	Trained nurse who contracted with a family to care for a sick family member in the home.
public health nurse	Also called district nurse, or visiting nurse. Worked outside of the hospital institution in the community with families of the sick poor and the middle class. As part of the early twentieth century public health movement, they taught preventive health care and preserved the health of people in the community as well as baby clinics, factories, schools, and shops.
trained nurse	Graduate of one-, two-, or three-year nurse training program.
graduate nurse	Replaced the term trained nurse.
registered nurse	Graduate nurse who successfully completed a state examination and met a minimum standard of practice acceptable in that particular state.
superintendent of nurse training school	The principal or directress of a nurse training school. Teaching, administration, and clinical supervision were among the responsibilities of the position.
superintendent	In many hospitals, the person responsible for the administration of nurses and training of student nurses.

Glossary

matron	In some hospitals, the person responsible for nurses and administration of nursing care in hospitals.
head nurse	Responsible for the supervision of a hospital ward. This position was usually held by second-year nursing students.
preliminary training course	An academic program that ranged from three weeks to five months needed to enhance the education provided by nurse training schools.
nursing registration	State credentialing of registered nurses.
post-graduate programs	Advanced nursing specialization programs that followed the two or three years of nurse training schools.

1

From Separate to Active Spheres

From its nature, nursing is peculiarly a woman's work . . . women have brought it to its present stage of development, and it is to women we must look for its future advancement.

Louise Darche, 1893[1]

DURING THE NINETEENTH century, American society saw nursing within the natural woman's role. Women served as the nurses in their own families and communities and within the public almshouses. Since no formal training for nurses existed prior to the 1870s, women learned nursing through apprenticeship and practice and few received payment for the care given. Women who nursed in almshouses were stereotyped as slovenly, unkempt, and immoral; many were drunkards, prisoners, or patients themselves. During the Civil War, women volunteers in the North and the South served as nurses. Their successful efforts in aiding the casualties of war led many to question the lack of trained nurses and adequate health care in America. Following the Civil War, women shared the societal expectation of improving conditions within the civilian almshouses and hospitals. They focused their attention on the English nurse and heroine of the Crimean War, Florence Nightingale (1820–1910), as the model for the emerging profession. Nightingale published her ideas about nursing and health and founded the preeminent nurse training program at St. Thomas Hospital in London in 1860. Her ideas of nursing and of nursing education served as the model for nurse-training programs in America after 1873.

During the nineteenth century, men were drawn away from their homes to urban jobs created in the industrialization of the American economy. Women, however, continued to work at home, providing care for their families. Reward for a woman's unpaid labor depended on her husband's or father's income and financial support. By the 1830s, men were earning wages and had gained political power while women earned praise and gained "moral superiority." For many women, this separation between men and women's roles was untenable and difficult to uphold. Although an avid supporter of women's separate sphere, Sarah Josepha Hale (1788–1879), editor of *Godey's Lady's Book* between 1837 and 1877, advanced the idea of women's education and women's professional roles. Pioneers opened seminaries and colleges for women's education. Women from upper and middle class families filled these schools and learned not only how to be better mothers and wives, but also how to teach. Curriculums in these schools offered women a wider range of subjects than previously available to women and thus prepared them to think and challenge societal norms.[2]

More liberal in their attitudes were those women involved in the nineteenth-century woman's movement. Women in this movement demanded equality in their political, social, and economic lives. Activists in the woman's movement formed associations demanding the right to vote and the right to speak. They claimed control of educational and financial opportunities for American women in women's sphere of domesticity as well as in the sphere of men in the world outside the home.[3]

Nursing as a profession began within this changing social climate. Women who pioneered nursing education in the late nineteenth century had to challenge women's roles as natural-born caregivers and had to overcome existing resistance to the professional role of nursing within the male-dominated institutions of almshouses and newly forming hospitals.[4]

Many events in America influenced changing women's roles and the transformation of accepted women's roles and the development of nursing as a profession during the nineteenth and early twentieth century. Contemporary ideas concerning women's roles, women's education and women's rights directly influenced the rise of the nursing profession during the nineteenth century. The developing nursing profession was influenced by as well as contributed to the ideology of domestic and social feminism of the late nineteenth and early twentieth century, and parallels emerged between nursing's growth as a profession and the prevailing ideas of women's rights to study, to work, and to vote.

WOMEN IN THE NINETEENTH CENTURY

In 1851, woman suffragist Elizabeth Cady Stanton (1815–1893) urged women to educate their girls toward "a life of self-dependence" and to prepare them "for some trade or profession."[5] Stanton pleaded for women's financial independence at a time in American history when most women were expected to stay at home, care for families, and depend on men for financial support. In nineteenth-century America, urbanization and industrialization had produced separate men and women's roles. A woman's "separate sphere" emerged as middle-class urban women cared for the home while their men attended to the business outside. Financial and social independence were traits not encouraged in girls or women in this changing industrial society. Instead, society primed women to care for family needs at home and to be responsible for the moral upbringing of children. Men, however, learned to function responsibly in the broader world of work, business, and politics. In antebellum America, few career opportunities for women existed beyond those within the accepted woman's domain. Women worked in the fields of "teaching, needle-work, keeping boarders, work in cotton mills, type-setting, book-binding, and household service."[6]

The element of time accentuated the separate spheres of men and women because the demands of industrialization and the movement of work from the home to the factory or office forced an adherence to artificial rather than natural time schedules. Weekly wages dictated that men's work be paid by the hour, while the unending series of unpredictably scheduled daily tasks at home continued to control the duration of woman's work. Her family's need to be fed and cared for governed the schedule of woman's unpaid labor at home.

Married men working outside the home expected to return home to a "safe harbor" and their wives, for the most part, accepted this expectation. Women's unpaid work contributed to the family's well-being, and thus was considered socially relevant. The idea of a virtuous womanhood, prevalent at the beginning of the nineteenth century, continued to shape the image of women's roles well into the twentieth century.[7] However, a paradox emerged as society glorified women's unpaid labor at home but demanded that men seek monetarily valued employment outside. Women's work at home was "idealized, yet rejected by men," resulting in what historian Nancy Cott characterizes as a "simultaneous glorification and devaluation."[8] Men demanded payment for their work and a political voice in a world that discouraged women from such expectation or participation. Women who accepted gender separation and stayed at home enjoyed the lauded status bestowed upon them, which nonetheless left them politically, socially, and economically dependent on men. Those women who challenged their second-class status in society faced opposition as they sought the vote, an education, and paid employment in a profession.[9]

Throughout the nineteenth century, the ideas of mainstream American society about education for women changed and expanded to include, as a necessity, education to guarantee women's successful fulfillment of their domestic tasks within woman's separate sphere of influence. An education for a woman as a future mother prepared her to guide the family's morality, rear the children properly, and manage an economically sound home. A wife became a non-threatening yet "more capable" adjunct to her husband.[10] During the Victorian era, women's education was established as an important component of the mainstream concept of the role of women. Although some schools offered coeducational opportunities for women, arguments favoring separate education for men and women prevailed. By the 1830s, a woman's education in the newly opened female seminaries prepared her for a teaching role. As a teacher she earned financial independence while remaining true to the bounds imposed upon her by society's prescribed woman's sphere. After the Civil War, the number of schools, both sex-segregated and coeducational, continued to increase and more women received an education suitable for the prescribed roles in society.[11]

Christian philosophy dominated each new women's academy and seminary as faculty educated women students to serve as America's future wives, mothers, and teachers. To achieve this, schools daily enforced structured routine, discipline, and prayer as well as the academic subjects of English, arithmetic, philosophy, geology, history, art, and language. Many of the new academies and seminaries developed innovative curriculums and included subjects such as mathematics, science, and physical education, previously taught only at men's schools. Pioneering women educators opened seminaries and colleges as a means of both financially supporting themselves and of improving other women's lives. Their visionary leadership and ideas carried many of these institutions forward into the twentieth century while continuing to serve as prototypes for future schools.

Emma Willard (1787–1870), one of the celebrated female educators of the early nineteenth century, opened the Troy Female Seminary in 1821. Willard had been a staunch advocate of public funding for women's schools and had published a plan in 1819 explaining her proposal, *An Address to the Public: Particularly to the Members of the Legislature of New York, Proposing a Plan for Improving Female Education.* Succeeding state legislatures rejected her plan to publicly fund women's education. However, a few years later, The Common Council of Troy, New York, offered to raise $40,000 to assist Willard to begin a school in their city. Accepting the offer, Willard created a financially successful private school for women. The expanded curriculum at the Troy Female Seminary offered women students more courses in liberal arts and sciences then had previously ever been available to them. At Troy they studied an extensive list of subjects including arithmetic, languages, trigonometry, and geography for the specific purpose of becoming adequately prepared teachers. By offering a richer academic curriculum, Willard pushed the frontier of women's education toward the outer boundaries of the prescribed woman's sphere. However, philosophically, her school reinforced those boundaries and prepared women to assume not only the role of teacher but their roles as wives and mothers as well.[12]

In May 1823, author and educator Catherine Beecher (1800–1878), began the Hartford Female Seminary for the daughters of the wealthy families in Hartford, Connecticut. As Hartford students, the girls received Beecher's evangelical preaching along with an education. Beecher envisioned her school as an endowed seminary and used her connections among the prestigious families in Hartford to obtain needed financial support. Her success at fund-raising enabled the school to move into new quarters with a staff of eight teachers in 1828. Her purpose in educating women stretched beyond that of refining young women. Beecher, like Willard, believed that an education should provide women an opportunity to be useful while staying within the bounds defined by the sphere of domesticity. Therefore, Beecher's Hartford Female Seminary educated women to teach. The curriculum reflected this goal by including a range of courses such a chemistry, using new equipment and textbooks, as well as courses focused on mental and moral philosophy.[13]

Two other women who opened seminaries during this period were Mary Lyons (1797–1849), and her friend and teacher, Zilpah Grant (1794–1874). Both women were greatly influenced by Reverend Joseph Emerson, the head of the Byfield Female Academy and avid supporter of advanced education for middle-class women. Drawing from their experiences at Byfield, Grant, with the help of Lyons, organized the Ipswich Female Seminary in 1829. Though successful in establishing its academic program, Grant and Lyons failed to secure a financial endowment for the school which closed in 1839. Mary Lyons, without Grant's help, however, focused on establishing an endowed school for women and continued to work towards her goal. Successfully soliciting support and donations from church women and other mothers of future students, Lyons opened the Mount Holyoke Female Seminary in South Hadley, Massachusetts in 1837. From the onset, Mt. Holyoke differed from other seminaries of the time because Lyons wanted women in the middle class to have an opportunity to attend school. Lyons made her Mount Holyoke affordable to middle-class families by reducing the school's operating costs. Instead of employing servants, Mt. Holyoke students performed all the domestic chores. Therefore, Lyons' students learned independence through a program of domestic duties, academic work, and physical exercise. Her success at Mount Holyoke often served as a model for future women seminaries and colleges that developed throughout the nineteenth century.[14]

In an attempt to institute a lasting memorial to himself, Matthew Vassar (1792–1858), created an innovative educational choice for women by founding Vassar College. Vassar Female College opened in 1865 (renamed Vassar College in 1867) and for the first time offered women a full collegiate liberal arts curriculum. Vassar distinguished itself as a women's college, rather than a women's seminary, by offering a broader curriculum than other women's schools and by supplying the proper equipment, environment, and faculty to successfully implement it. Concerned about criticism of the effect of its innovative collegiate plan on developing young women, Vassar incorporated the homelike structure of the seminary into his college. Students lived together with the few un-married female faculty in one building rather than in small separate pavilions reserved for the male faculty and their families. The president, John H. Raymond, former head of the Collegiate and Polytechnic Institute in Brooklyn, paternally supervised the college while the lady principal, Hannah Lyman, formerly from Ipswich Academy, offered a maternal influence.[15]

In 1875, Henry Fowle Durant (1822–1881), a prominent lawyer who became a preacher and trustee at Mt. Holyoke, opened the next women's college in Wellesley, Massachusetts. Like the earlier women's seminary, Mt. Holyoke, Wellesley College hoped to educate women to serve as teachers. However, Durant viewed college as women's salvation from the subordinate position they held in society. Durant hired a female faculty for Wellesley and set a precedent for future women board members by appointing his wife, Pauline Durant, as a college trustee. He also selected a woman, Ada Howard, a Mt. Holyoke graduate, as Wellesley's first president. Durant envisioned college as a medium for his religious beliefs and required each faculty member and trustee to be a member of an evangelical church. He continued to preach at the school and instituted Bible studies, chapel services, and quiet devotions into the daily routine. Attracted to the design of its predecessor, Vassar College, Durant built an architecturally beautiful college that provided an elegant surrounding for the college life that he envisioned for women students.[16]

Smith College, the first women's college to be endowed by a woman, was opened in 1975 by Sophia Smith (1796–1870), who bequeathed the sum of $393,105 to the school in Northampton, Massachusetts. Through the help of Amherst professors William Seymour Tyler (1810–1897), and Julius Hawley Seelye (1824–1895), Smith donated the funds that enabled women to receive a collegiate education comparable to existing men's colleges. An evangelical religious spirit pervaded the college curriculum that Smith requested in her will. Smith believed that women receiving such an education would be better prepared to reform the evils found in society. She emphasized that education expanded women's usefulness within their roles as mothers, teachers, and writers. Smith's first president, the Reverend Laurenus Clark Seelye (1873–1910), furthered Sophia Smith's ideas during the school's formative years.

Prior to the opening of Smith College, L. Clark Seelye gave several speeches on the subject of women's education in order to add additional funds to Smith's legacy. He strongly advocated educating women in women's colleges and argued that coeducation had not improved the morality of male students at coed schools as had been anticipated. Nor did he believe that women enrolled in existing coeducational schools demonstrated an intellect inferior or superior to men.[17]

Seelye supported single-sex schools because women and men could fully develop and refine their distinctive traits attributed to the specific sex in such schools. Seelye argued his point of view by refuting an analogy commonly used by coeducational supporters that if you plant a pine tree and rose bush together in the same soil, both would grow as a pine tree and rose bush. What if the soil favored the pine tree's growth, Seelye asked, *then* the rose bush would wither. He related this to women's education by asking, "What if the same forces which develop all that is most manly in one sex repress and dwarf all that is most womanly in the other?"[18] Seelye saw college as more than a means of defining and preparing a woman's usefulness. A woman needed a broader education than the one that simply prepared her for her work, the same way a man needed a broader education than one that prepared him only for his occupation or career.

Seelye designed the school differently than previous women's seminaries and colleges. He wanted to maintain a homelike atmosphere that did not socially isolate students from town or from men. Instead of the strict rules of conduct and ringing bells that ordered the life of students at other women's colleges, Smith students were free to decide their daily schedule and their social lives. The school believed that daily chapel, classes, gymnastics, meals, and a "student's sense of decorum"[19] were sufficient to regulate the students' life. No escorts were needed to accompany Smith students on their walks, rides, or other activities that brought them into contact with people in the nearby town of Northampton, Massachusetts. The design of the school conformed to Seelye's wish for a homelike setting. Its buildings consisted of one large structure for classrooms and administration and smaller, separate cottages for students to live in. A female faculty member and a "lady-in-charge" lived in each of the student residences. Sophia Smith provided the financial foundation for the college while Reverend L. Clark Seelye provided the school's philosophical underpinnings. Their commitment and vision converged to establish Smith College as another step toward women's equal opportunity for advanced education.[20]

Other important women's schools opened during the latter quarter of the nineteenth century. The founder of Bryn Mawr, Joseph Wright Taylor, started his school for women in 1884. It offered an advanced curriculum enriched by an Orthodox Quaker context. However, what made Bryn Mawr unique among the early women's colleges was the contribution of its first dean and second president, M. Carey Thomas (1857–1935). Under her energetic and charismatic leadership, Bryn Mawr demanded a standard of rigorous academic excellence of Bryn Mawr students that equalled that of men's colleges.

Thomas achieved academic excellence from her students by setting stringent admission requirements similar to those of Harvard University. Among her students she enforced a stringent academic discipline that remained in place until her retirement in 1922. A feminist and suffragist, Thomas ardently supported women's rights and she shared these views with her students and with a larger audience when she became first president of the National College Women's Equal Suffrage League in 1908. Thomas earned Bryn Mawr a reputation as an elite women's college that challenged both a woman's intellect and a woman's role in society. Showing foresight and initiative, M. Carey Thomas authorized the opening in 1921 of the influential Bryn Mawr Summer School for Women Workers, a school for labor activist education dedicated to blue collar and organized labor women.[21]

Barnard College, another important school for women, opened in 1889 at Columbia University in New York City after much debate over the merits of higher education for women. Columbia's first experiment at women's education began in 1883 with the start of the Columbia Collegiate Course for Women. In this first attempt, Columbia gave an entrance exam and periodic exams to women over a four-year period. Those who passed the exams received a degree at the end of the four years. However, few women applied for the program because the college provided no instruction to women. Annie Nathan Meyer (1867–1951), successfully entered Columbia's Collegiate Course for Women in 1885 and stayed until 1887 when she married. She argued against the barring of women from lectures and fought to open a women's college at Columbia. Seeking independent patrons and recruiting the help of Mary Mapes Dodge (1831–1905), Ella Weed

(1853–1894), and Melvil Dewey (1851–1931), Meyer successfully obtained the signatures of fifty prominent New Yorkers to support her idea. The new college was to be named after the recently deceased Frederick Augustus Porter Barnard (1809–1889), president of Columbia University and avid supporter of coeducation. Ella Weed served on its board of trustees and as chairman of Barnard's academic committee.

In Barnard's formative years, women students received the same entrance exams as the students at Columbia. Those who passed attended classes in converted brownstones on Madison Avenue and Forty-Ninth Street in New York City. Unlike other women's colleges, many of Barnard's urban students commuted daily to classes rather than experiencing the cloistered campus life of other residential schools. Barnard's early curriculum offered students mathematics, Latin, Greek, English, and German. In order to add his philosophy course to the Barnard curriculum, Nicholas Murray Butler (1862–1947) had first to change Columbia's bylaws. By including Barnard women in his course at Columbia, Butler saved both time from teaching two separate courses and the cost to Barnard of duplicating his course. Barnard needed to raise additional money in order for the school to build and to continue. Three financial backers, Mrs. Van Wyck Brickerhoff, Mrs. Elizabeth Milbank Anderson, and Mrs. Josiah W. Fiske, endowed the first three buildings designed specifically for the college. Another woman, Emily O. Gibbes, provided Barnard with its first large endowment gift.[22]

The educational landscape for women changed again with the opening of Radcliffe College in 1894 at Harvard University. Radcliffe was unique among the women's colleges because of its relationship with Harvard College. Beginning in 1873, twenty-seven women, in a newly formed organization called "The Society for the Collegiate Instruction of Women," studied together with Harvard College professors. Known as the Annex, this group served as the forerunner of Radcliffe College. Unlike other women's colleges which possessed their own faculties, Radcliffe continued the practice, started by the Annex, of having women study with the male faculty at Harvard. Another fundamental difference between Radcliffe and the other women's colleges was that its granting of the bachelor of arts degree required a co-signature from Harvard.[23]

In the nineteenth century, most women college students attended the increasing number of single-sex seminaries and colleges. However, some attended the few coeducational opportunities available to them. Oberlin in 1833 provided one of the earliest coeducational experiences. While still upholding women's moral responsibility and separate role, women earned undergraduate degrees for the first time. Other coeducational schools followed, such as Swarthmore in 1864 and Cornell University in 1877. Throughout the midwest, land-grant colleges were added to these coeducational institutions that offered women opportunities to advance their education. Although some coeducational schools educated women to comply with society's acceptable sphere of domesticity, many of these schools expanded their curriculums to areas of study and thought previously denied to women.[24]

Women's education, and specifically the founding of women's schools, received support from Sarah Josepha Hale (1788–1879), editor of the influential periodical, *Godey's Lady's Book*. Hale's monthly editorials asked the public to support the growth of women's schools and urged legislators to fund such schools equally with those of men. Unsuccessful at obtaining public funding, Hale encouraged wealthy patrons to financially support the new women's schools. Her editorials endorsed new curriculums at women's schools that were to educate America's new and upcoming teachers. The religious overtones in these schools complemented Hale's ideas of women's piety and morality. Hale saw women's higher education and entry into the teaching profession as the means to the "improvement of her sex" and the elevated spirituality of her nation. These schools offered their students an opportunity to learn within a framework of acceptable domesticity. Women could improve their minds and their lives without overtly challenging the gender role society had dictated for them. Hale's conservatism encouraged women to stretch the boundaries of women's sphere but not to step beyond them. Although a staunch advocate of advanced education for women, Hale did not lend her support to woman's suffrage. Not alone in this predilection, other strong proponents of women's education such as Emma Willard, Catherine Beecher, and Mary Lyons shared a philosophy that stopped short of advocating women's equality to men.[25]

Developed by twentieth-century historian Daniel Scott Smith, the term "domestic feminism" has been used to describe the focused advocacy of many of these antebellum women writers and educators who promoted women's education and an expanded definition of women's work while continuing to believe that women should stay within the defined sphere of domesticity. These nineteenth-century educators opened institutions where women received an education and transformed teaching into a woman's profession. Women educated in these schools learned how to teach the academics and at the same time learned to save souls. They stayed within the bounds of domesticity, yet paved the way for other women to challenge the closed boundaries of women's separate sphere.[26]

Nineteenth-century American society sanctioned education for women because better educated women made better mothers, wives, and teachers. However, some of the nineteenth century's better educated women questioned the lack of formal training for nursing and of the professionalism of the caring role that women had previously "naturally" assumed. Although the newly formed nineteenth-century American seminaries may have educated women to be morally superior and better teachers, these institutions did not prepare women for the demands made on them as they worked as nurses in the home or later as nurses on the battlefields during the Civil War (1861–1865). First the Crimean War (1854–1857), and then the Civil War in America, exposed the glaringly unsafe and unsanitary health care conditions on the battlefields. In both wars, women for the first time were permitted to serve as nurses in military medical facilities to care for wounded soldiers. Their life-saving work in remedying the squalid conditions of war led many social reformers to attempt the reform of civilian hospitals. It became apparent to many women that just as education prepared teachers to save souls, education for nurses would prepare them to save lives.

THE MODERN NURSING MOVEMENT

After the 1850s, the modern nursing movement offered women a career opportunity other than teaching. This movement started in the late 1850s following Florence Nightingale's (1820–1910) work in the Crimean War and provided women opportunities to study the art and science of nursing in newly forming nurse training schools in America. As the founder of this movement, Nightingale influenced the growth of nursing education in America and throughout the world. The movement grew in response to her reforms in Great Britain, including the application of sanitary science in hospitals, the use of trained nurses in military and civilian hospitals, and the demand for education of nurses.[27]

Nightingale informed the public of unsafe conditions that she found in hospitals and described her philosophy and theory of nursing through her many publications such as the highly acclaimed *Notes on Nursing; What it is, and What it is not,* first published in 1859. She statistically linked poor sanitary conditions of hospitals to increased death rates of patients and further established the role of nursing in improving these conditions. She wrote that, ". . . there is some fear lest hospitals, as they have been *hitherto,* may not have generally increased, rather than diminished, the rate of mortality . . ."[28]

Nightingale argued that women who studied nursing must learn and apply the laws of health to the well person to prevent illness. However, this was difficult because "the very elements of what constitutes good nursing are as little understood for the well as for the sick."[29] In her *Notes on Nursing,* Nightingale detailed for the reader her ideas of what composed the laws of health and how to care for the sick. According to her biographer, Sir Edward Cook:

> *Miss Nightingale was the founder of modern nursing because she made public opinion perceive, and act upon the perception, that nursing was an art, and must be raised to the status of a trained profession.*[30]

The ideas of Florence Nightingale and of trained nurses influenced the growth of hospitals as health care institutions from the mid-nineteenth to the early twentieth century.[31] Hospitals during the pre-industrialization era in America primarily provided custodial care for the ill rather than dramatic medical cures. Usually run as charitable institutions or religious organizations, these institutions provided some form of nursing care along with limited medical treatment. According to medical historian Paul Starr, a typical medical practitioner at the turn of the nineteenth century may have spent an entire career without ever stepping into a hospital. However, hospitals during the nineteenth century underwent change as a result of the Industrial Revolution. During this period, people moved to the city to find work, lived in smaller quarters, and had less time to care for their sick at home. Those who typically stayed at home and cared for the sick found their caregiving role dramatically altered by the changes in work habits, home-life, and family roles that the new industrial society produced. People needing health care often found themselves alone and removed from the physical and emotional support of their families. Simultaneously, hospitals became safer places to survive an illness as a result of sanitary reforms implemented by educated nurses and advances in germ theory used in medicine to invoke new cures; thus, the hospital staff slowly replaced the patient's "family" in the care of the ill.[32]

Until nurse training programs began in the 1870s, ambulatory patients, untrained attendants, or members of religious orders administered nursing care in hospitals. Untrained women, often on loan from local almshouses, also worked in hospitals performing needed domestic duties. Contemporary historian Charles Rosenberg expands upon the stereotypical image of the nurse during the antebellum period, explaining that both men and women served as nurses, and not all were "recruited among the depraved and infirmed."[33] However, many of the untrained attendants and nurses were considered to be unsavory characters likened in many nursing histories to Charles Dickens's fictional Sairey Gamp.[34]

The sanitary reforms implemented by Nightingale provided patients with pure air, proper ventilation, nutritious food, and improved sanitary conditions in hospitals and homes. Nightingale's insistence that nurses needed to undergo a formal training program significantly transformed hospitals into safer environments for patients. Along with Nightingale's sanitary reforms and nurse training, the introduction of the germ theory and other late nineteenth-century scientific discoveries further "cleaned" up the hospital. People began to see hospitals as places of healing rather than of dying. At the same time, physicians in the newly established medical profession were finding that hospitals were becoming safer places in which to practice medicine.

Prior to the Civil War, anyone could claim to be a nurse. Women's duty to nurse their families and the sick fit within the natural boundary prescribed by women's separate sphere. A woman relied on apprenticeship and her innate abilities to learn the necessary things one had to know in order to keep her family healthy. "Born" into her nursing role, formal education seemed superfluous and unnecessary. Women learned what they needed to know from each other, and hospital administrators reinforced this idea by using untrained, unskilled women in their institutions. Some of these women nursed better than others, but the quality of care they provided was unsupervised, unregulated, and unsafe.

For the most part, wherever possible, care of the sick continued to be provided in the home rather than in the charitable hospitals of that period, and typically women in the home performed that task. Because it was considered women's duty, women learned from each other the needed skills to care for the family's health.[35]

At the outbreak of the Civil War in 1861, there were few, if any, trained nurses available to meet the needs of the country. Thus, an estimated 2,000 women, self-taught volunteers, "born nurses," and "practical motherly nurses" provided nursing care throughout the war in military and civilian hospitals.[36] High mortality rates in hospitals existed due to the unsanitary conditions found in them. Nevertheless, civilian hospitals tried to meet the increased demand the war placed on nursing care as did Catholic and Protestant religious orders opening their hospitals to accommodate those who needed care.

Physician Elizabeth Blackwell (1821–1910) contributed significantly to the formation of the United States Sanitary Commission, originally organizing volunteers to be sent to Bellevue Hospital in New York City for a brief nurse training period. The sanitary commission, established June 9, 1861, grew from the auxiliary, The Woman's Central Relief Association, founded by Louisa Lee Schuyler (1837–1927) during April of the same year. The sanitary commission provided supplies and relief to soldiers throughout the Civil War and relied on the volunteerism of women to raise money, improve sanitary conditions, nurse the wounded, and provide moral support to those who fought the war. Aware of Nightingale's success, members of the sanitary commission consulted Nightingale to learn how she had improved the quality of nursing care and the conditions that she found in the military hospitals of the Crimea.[37]

In recounting the sanitary commission's outstanding work, author Frank Moore in 1866 reported that for every soldier who died on the battlefield, two died from disease. This statistic, he wrote, demonstrated an improvement over the mortality rate of the Crimean War, in which seven-eighths died from disease and one-eighth died from battle wounds. Moore attributed to the "labors and sacrifices by our loyal women" a saving of more than 184,000 men who would have died as a result of malaria, exposure of the filth of the camps, infection from the hospital conditions, and depression.[38]

At the close of the Civil War, the vivid experiences of the untrained volunteer nurses on the battlefields influenced many social activists to consider education for nurses essential.[39] America witnessed Nightingale's early success in nursing education at her newly established training school which opened June 24, 1860, in London's St. Thomas Hospital. The Nightingale Fund, founded by the English in honor of Florence Nightingale after the Crimean War, provided the initial funds for the school. The first class at St. Thomas started with fifteen women who lived, worked, and studied together at the hospital. Called probationers, these new students received instruction in the art and science of nursing from the experienced nurses at St. Thomas's hospital (called sisters), as well as lectures on disease from the medical staff. As part of their training, students worked as assistant nurses and were graded according to technical ability and a good moral record. Students lived together on one of the upper floors of St. Thomas with two sisters who were responsible for them. Probationers each received their own room, board, uniforms and ten pounds for personal expenses. As a prerequisite for admission, students brought with them character references which helped the school meet its goal of improving the character of each new probationer. The matron of the school, Mrs. Wardroper, supervised the probationers' education and moral development and supplied discipline when needed. Thirteen of the first fifteen probationers completed the first year "experiment" at St. Thomas, thus establishing the model for future schools of nursing throughout the world.[40]

Nightingale's belief that women should control the teaching and practice of nursing was revolutionary. She maintained this feminist stance in the face of opposition from paternalistic physicians and hospital boards who wished to exercise control of nursing's future education. Although some supported nurse training at that time, "the medical profession as a whole was unsympathetic or hostile towards reforms . . ."[41] A 1908 editorial appearing in *The American Journal of Nursing (AJN)* explained that:

> *Miss Nightingale's . . . brilliant essence lay in her taking from men's hands a power which did not logically or rightly belong to them, but which they had usurped, and seizing it firmly in her own, from whence she passed it on to her pupils and disciples. In this she was a glorious and successful revolutionary.*[42]

Sir Edward Cook believed that Nightingale recognized that her pioneering work directly related to the woman's movement.[43] For the first time, newly established nursing schools formally prepared nurses according to a model of education set by the Nightingale School at St. Thomas's Hospital. These trained Nightingale nurses, as envisioned by Nightingale, scattered throughout the world and helped to establish modern schools of nursing in America.[44]

In the post-Civil War period in the United States, the impetus to open professional training schools for nurses came from public-minded women, many of whom had volunteered during the Civil War in hospitals and in activities of the United States Sanitary Commission. Their efforts to open nurse training schools also encountered strong opposition from the male-dominated medical profession which obstructed but did not deter the supporters of professional nursing training.[45]

Prior to the Civil War, the few attempts by physicians, often women physicians, to educate secular women in the art of nursing met with little public recognition or lasting success. The first training school for nurses was started in New York in 1798 by an attending physician at New York Hospital, Valentine Seaman. Seaman organized a course of lectures for nurses that ranged from anatomy and physiology to midwifery and child care. Philadelphian physician Joseph Warrington, with the help of Philadelphia's Quaker community, began to train nurses when he founded the Philadelphia Lying-in Charity in 1828. Warrington included in his course the subject of midwifery. In hopes of attracting students and combating a shortage of applicants, Warrington in 1839, and again in 1855, published leaflets describing his courses. Six years later, in 1861, also in Philadelphia, physician Ann Preston (1813–1872) founded The Woman's Hospital and opened a nurse training school. In this school, female physicians gave lectures to the nursing students. However, because of the Civil War, Preston's school did not fully develop until 1872 when the school, after a substantial financial endowment, was reorganized.[46]

In New York City, another physician "intimately acquainted" with Florence Nightingale, Elizabeth Blackwell, prepared to open what might have been America's first Nightingale-influenced nurse training school at her hospital, the New York Infirmary of Women and Children. Similar to the situation with the Woman's Hospital in Philadelphia, the Civil War prevented Blackwell from opening her school. However, another physician, Dr. Marie Zakrzewska (1829–1902), successfully founded one of the first training schools in America at the

New England Hospital for Women and Children. First chartered in 1862, the school did not open until September 1872. Linda Richards (1841–1930), became distinguished as America's first graduate nurse when she successfully completed the school's one-year course in nursing and received a certificate.[47]

The first three schools directly modeled after Nightingale's school at St. Thomas's opened in America in 1873. Women activists influenced the establishment of each of these schools. In New York City, the Bellevue Training School for Nurses opened in May of 1873 at Bellevue Hospital. Later that year, the New Haven Hospital in New Haven, Connecticut, opened the Connecticut Training School for Nurses. The third school, the Boston Training School for Nurses, began at Massachusetts General Hospital. Both the Bellevue Training School for Nurses and the Boston Training School for Nurses resulted from the "initiative of women . . . who sought ways to advance women and prepare them for self-support."[48] A committee of physicians at the New Haven Hospital started a nurse training school and formed a training school board composed of both men and women to assist in the process.[49]

Louisa Lee Schuyler (1837–1926), philanthropist and activist in the Woman's Central Association of Relief, initiated the Nightingale-modeled training school for nurses at Bellevue Hospital.[50] The bleak conditions in the city hospitals in New York, particularly Bellevue, led Schuyler in 1872 to organize the New York State Charities Association. The association formed a visiting committee to assess the conditions in the city's charitable institutions. The committee found that nurses at Bellevue, prior to the opening of the training school, were often prisoners, vagrants, and paupers from the nearby workhouse on Blackwell's Island. It learned of the rats that ran throughout the hospital, and of patients unattended at night who relied on untrained watchmen to call the doctor. As a result of its findings, the committee concluded that the only way to change the unhealthy conditions found at the hospital was to establish a training school for nurses. Prior to opening the school in 1873, W. Gill Wylie, a physician, visited Nightingale's school at St. Thomas's in England for guidance. Due to illness, Nightingale could not see him, but she wrote a detailed letter about her ideas regarding nursing education. The advice given in Nightingale's letter was the underpinning for the Bellevue school.[51]

Founders of Bellevue's training school recognized the advantages of recruiting educated women into nurse training and proposed "to train intelligent women to become skilled hospital nurses . . . thus improving hospital training not only at Bellevue, but throughout the country."[52] Those who completed and graduated from one of the newly formed schools became known as trained nurses. Trained nurses, later referred to as "graduate nurses," became the next generation of nursing leaders and educators, as well as the rank and file nurses in hospitals and homes throughout America. Nursing educator Isabel Maitland Stewart (1878–1963) asserted that the modern nursing movement trained and educated women into "spheres of action."[53] She further maintained that nurse training schools served" . . . the purpose of making women socially useful outside of the domestic sphere, emancipating them and giving them a chance to grow."[54]

Nursing educators challenged the limited sphere of domesticity and extended the previously conceived "natural role" of women as nurses into one that required training and education. However, the conflicting missions of the new schools of nursing—to educate women in the art and science of nursing or to train cheap workers to provide hospital service, often created confusion as to what the graduates were. Images of nurses as conjured by use of the interchangeable terms "trained" or "educated" created some ambiguity in the understanding of the public. Whether trained or educated, nurses learned certain ". . . fundamental principles, discriminating observation and judgement, appreciation of values, ethical ideals, a high sense of responsibility, capacity for initiative and loyal co-operation." Once trained or educated, nurses possessed the ability to ". . . investigate health conditions and use statistical data" in their clinical practice. However, confusion stemmed from whether the central goal of hospital schools was to provide a charitable service to patients or professional education for nurses. In either case, nurse training was not supposed to produce ". . . an automaton or a routineer."[55]

In some respects, use of the term "trained nurses" hampered the profession in the thirty years following the founding of the first school of nursing. Isabel Hampton Robb (1860–1910), first president of the Nurses' Associated Alumnae, which formed in 1896, believed that the public associated "training" with mechanical rather than intellectual development of nursing. Both aspects, she argued, were important to the growing profession of nursing. Unfortunately when the nineteenth-century public heard the term "nurse," it thought of either the slovenly Sairey Gamp or the child's nurse or nanny. The public was not sure whether these newly trained nurses were educated to think or trained to serve. Thus, in order to move nursing out of the private sphere of domesticity and into a public sphere of action, nurse educators had to contend with the tensions created between the perceived image of nursing and the increasingly demanding educational process required of this emerging profession. As a result of the improved nursing care in hospitals that had training schools, the public recognized that in either case, some formal preparation for nurses had an educative and practical value.[56]

Some of the newly formed schools graduated trained nurses within a one-year training period, while others added an additional year of hospital service to their curriculum. Following successful completion of the second year of training, students were granted diplomas as public recognition of their service to the school.[57] By the early 1890s, most schools had adopted a two-year course; after 1893, visionary nursing leaders were advocating a three-year program to provide uniform curriculum and shorter work days for the students. However, this expansion of the curriculum to meet the educational needs of nurse training evolved slowly. For example, by 1900 the extended three-year course was found in only 137 out of 433 nurse training schools in the United States.[58]

Those hospitals that started a nurse training program found a cheap labor source in the "pupil nurse." Students, rather than paid graduate nurses, staffed their hospital wards. Some graduates with executive abilities were hired to supervise and teach the pupil nurses, but once they completed their nurse training, most graduate nurses were forced to become independent wage-earners and worked as private duty nurses who contracted to care for sick patients at home. Training schools sometimes maintained a nursing registry to help their graduates find private duty jobs outside the hospital.[59]

Prior to 1893, before the first professional nursing organization formed, there was no uniformity in curriculum among the new nurse training schools. The first year of nurse training often consisted of sixteen to twenty-four hours of physicians' lectures on various theoretical topics supplemented by practical instruction "at the bedside" by the head nurse and physician. Instructors paid little attention to the sequencing of the topics, which varied from year to year and from school to school. Topics of lectures listed in a Bellevue report in 1875 included, "Food for children and treatment of the child after birth," "The eye," "The wonderful discoveries of the ophthalmoscope," "A breath of fresh air," "What to do in emergencies," "Digestion and food," "Testing urine," "Circulation," "Surgical instruments and preparation for operation," "Bandaging," "Symptoms of disease," "Puerperal women," "Medicines," "Inflammation," and "Haemorrhage."[60]

Pupil nurses in their first year of training could be called on to fill head nurse positions on the hospital wards whenever a scarcity of new graduates existed. Louise Darche (1852–1899), superintendent of the Training School for Nurses on Blackwell's Island in New York City, found that by extending nurse training to two years, students would acquire enough practical knowledge to be ". . . retained and utilized as head nurses" in the second.[61]

Between 1870 and 1920, the number of single, financially self-supporting, and in some instances, liberally educated women increased. New opportunities arose in which to broaden woman's sphere from private domesticity to public activity because of the Woman's Rights movement. Women expressed interest in improving social conditions in America and branched off in many directions, joining women's clubs, suffrage organizations, and settlement houses to do this. The needs of women coincided with the needs of the emerging profession of nursing in the late nineteenth and early twentieth century. The newly formed nurse training schools recruited older and more mature "respectable women" as students, while such women searched for a respectable, paid occupation in which to support themselves. The number of schools increased to meet the rising demand of new applicants who sought professional training. Between 1873 and 1880, fifteen training schools had opened in the United States and had granted diplomas to 323 trained nurses. By 1900, the number of schools rose to 422 and the number of graduates to more than 11,000.[62]

In the 1900 United States Census, graduate nurses were distinguished by category from untrained nurses, who were referred to as practical or domestic nurses. Census figures indicate that nurse training schools were making inroads in providing the public with better prepared nurses; in 1900, there were 11,804 graduate nurses; in 1910, 82,327; and in 1920, 149,128. The number of graduate nurses had increased from 16 nurses per 100,000 population in 1900 to 141 nurses per 100,000 population in 1920. The number of untrained nurses rose from 13,483 to 151,996 in 1920, bringing an almost equal number of trained and untrained nurses into the public domain.[63]

The nursing profession simultaneously afforded American women a means of fulfilling their designated role of service to society and an opportunity to be self-supporting. Both fitted within the acceptable woman's sphere and as such should not have been threatening to men. Just as women's work in the home was glorified and the wife was considered a non-threatening auxiliary to her husband, nursing offered a parallel professional role to the practice of medicine. Trained nurses were to be the physician's "nonthreatening" assistants while providing a safe "home" for the patient within the hospital. Thus, this modern nursing movement, which trained nurses to be self-sufficient and disciplined as well as gentle and compassionate, presumably did not represent any threat to the male-dominated society.[64]

In spite of the nursing profession's presumed subordinate nature, nurse educators and administrators have continually confronted the issue of who controlled the developing profession of nursing since the opening of training schools in 1873. In attempting to control the development, women in nursing challenged the idealized vision of a gentle, obedient female who nursed the sick. They argued with those who politically dominated the newly emerging hospitals—physicians and hospital administrators—for control of nursing students, the nursing school's curriculum, and nursing practice. Although Nightingale laid the groundwork for nurses to control nursing's professional evolution in training schools and hospital wards, proponents of American nursing faced a constant struggle. A report published in 1928 by the Committee of Grading Schools, which studied nursing's relationship with medicine, documented this persistent issue. The report noted that while medicine and nursing benefited from an exchange of professional knowledge and curriculum, nurses were never quite as interested in medical education as physicians were in nursing education. Physicians worried that nurses might become too independent, too educated, and too theoretical to serve as professional subordinates to the paternalistic physician's patients, "his" hospital, or "his" profession.[65]

From the outset of the modern nursing movement, Nightingale wanted to recruit women who were willing and capable of learning the art and science of nursing. Those who selected nursing did so as a professional choice and not because they were required to do so or in reaction to a previous romantic failure. Nightingale tried to dispel the popular notion that only women who had experienced a heartbreaking disappointment in life would select nurses as a means of forgetting their troubles and hopefully becoming heroines in the process. The "true spirit of learning," Nightingale said, did not stem from "a disgust to everything or something else."[66] She reasoned that the art of nursing was important enough to require sufficient learning and experience so that nurses could properly administer to patients and hospital wards. Nightingale advised women to select a profession based on their interests rather than on the dictates of society. She opposed equally the popular sentiment that directed women to select a profession because it was women's work.[67] She asked that her "sisters" avoid the use of the popular arguments promoted by women's rights activists which, according to Nightingale, encouraged women to choose a profession engaged in by men, like medicine, "merely because men do it," and not because it suited them better. She held the same views toward arguments which urged "women to do nothing that men do, merely because they are women. . . ." Nightingale wanted women to be recognized for what they did and not whether it was "suitable" for them to do it. Gender should be eliminated as the criterion for the work that women did and women needed to ignore the external social cues which directed women into one career and men into another.

Nightingale envisioned the control of nursing in the hands of capable, educated women who selected nursing by choice and not by default. The newly opened training schools of the late nineteenth century offered American women the choice of a profession which allowed them to use their presumed traits of gentleness, compassion, and caring, as well as their ideas, knowledge, and abilities. The rise of nursing as a profession coincided with that of domestic feminism, when women expanded their lives from the private sphere into the public forum without destroying the existing gender system. The intent of early nursing pioneers like Florence Nightingale challenged the limited boundaries of women's work and may have equally questioned the assumption of the moral superiority of women's work, a viewpoint held by domestic feminists. Nightingale wrote, "it does not make a thing good, that it is remarkable that a woman should have been able to do it. Neither does it make a thing bad, which would have been good had a man done it, that it has been done by a woman."[68]

During the latter half of the nineteenth century and the beginning of the twentieth century, women's groups formed to address inequities found in society. Under the heading of social feminism, women worked through different organizations to improve social conditions in America for the urban poor, the immigrant labor force, and for women. Municipalities with a plethora of social ills offered women a "large house" to keep clean and healthy. Women approached such environments as occasions for their social housekeeping activities. A public health nurse and founder of the Henry Street Settlement in 1893, Lillian Wald recalled the social reform activities of women whose anger stemmed from confronting the unsanitary and unsightly mounds of manure found on city streets and prompted their social agitation that resulted in legislation which literally cleaned the streets:

> *One day in 1884 eleven women came together and decided to organize for the protection of the view and to improve the air by removing accumulations of manure which were piled up in the vicinity . . . they went up to Albany and a bill was introduced which made it a misdemeanor to have such accumulations within the city limits.*[69]

By the early twentieth century, organizations like the Association of Collegiate Alumnae, the General Federation of Club Women, the Woman's Christian Temperance Union, the National American Woman Suffrage Association, the National Consumers' League, and the National Women's Trade Union League had formed and implemented their progressive agendas. Forerunners of the chapters of the General Federation of Women's Clubs, local women's clubs formed immediately following the Civil War for this purpose. The activities of such clubs harnessed the energy of educated middle-class women who advocated the advance of women's education, work, and rights while still retaining the culture of a woman's separate sphere.[70]

Women in the newly emerging profession of nursing faced the same issues and interests that other women faced during the late nineteenth century and early twentieth century. The goals and interests of social feminists matched many of those in nursing who saw their profession as a means of improving the health of society. Nurse training, itself a result of woman's social-minded concern, further qualified nurses as participants in reform activities.[71] The nursing organizations which formed during the late nineteenth century differed from other organized women's groups because for the first time, women organized for professional growth and control. Nurses applied social feminist activism to their own professional needs to ensure the health of society. They saw the political connection between the issues of improved health for society and their own political involvement. Baltimore nurse and suffragist Mary Bartlett Dixon (1873–1957) argued that "our health . . . the quality and quantity of air in towns, homes, hospitals, stores and factories; our water, milk, food and drug supplies; the sewage and garbage questions, are all directly controlled by government."[72]

Nursing, as shown in Chapter Two, formed national and international associations. The purpose for these associations stemmed from nurses needing to defend, expand, and improve their occupation as professionals within the too often resistant and male-dominated medical establishments. Nurses struggled for professional equality amidst institutions that wanted nurses to stay within the circumscribed bounds of women's roles, specifically the limited role of caring.

The woman suffrage movement, through which women demanded the right to vote, preceded the modern nursing movement. During the era that extended from the antebellum period into the twentieth century, nursing became a bona fide profession as women argued for and later won the right to vote. Better educated and more informed during this period, women agitated for their political freedom. Early organizations within the suffrage movement set precedents that later women's groups followed. Nursing's subsequent organization into professional groups coincided with the increasingly political activities of the suffrage movement, hence, the profession of nursing found itself embroiled in the argument for woman suffrage.[73]

THE WOMAN SUFFRAGE MOVEMENT

The woman suffrage movement began in 1848 at the first organized Woman's Rights Convention held at Seneca Falls, New York, on the 19th and 20th of July. During that convention, Elizabeth Cady Stanton, Lucretia Mott (1793–1880), and several other women wrote the *Declaration of Sentiments,* which clearly affirmed their belief that,

". . . all men and women are created equal."[74] Modeled after the *Declaration of Independence,* the *Declaration of Sentiments* demanded an equal vote for women, an idea deemed too advanced for some in the antebellum woman's rights movement.[75]

As it had on the modern nursing movement, the Civil War had a great impact on the woman's rights movement. The abolitionist and woman's rights movements shared similar ideas and supporters during the antebellum period. Abolitionists focused on the emancipation of African-American slaves regardless of gender. However, as concerned for human freedom as the abolitionists seemed, not all supported a woman's right to vote, regardless of color. Consequently, when freedom finally came to the slave, only freedmen were enfranchised. Formerly enslaved by color, African-American women found themselves now enslaved by gender. As a freed slave, suffragist, abolitionist, and nurse during the Civil War, Sojourner Truth (1797–1883) frequently and eloquently spoke on behalf of woman suffrage. Truth delivered a speech in Akron, Ohio, in 1851 in which she responded to a heckler in the audience whose anti-suffrage stance regarded women as dependent and privileged. Truth rebutted this assertion, arguing that she had "ploughed, and planted, and gathered into barns . . . ," she had "borne thirteen children, and seen 'em, mos' all sold off to slavery" and yet as she repeatedly asked the audience "a'n't I a woman?" When Truth finished, the listeners applauded her speech "with streaming eyes and hearts beating with gratitude."[76]

The ratification of the Fourteenth Amendment on July 28, 1868, separated woman suffrage activists and members of the American Equal Rights Association (AERA), because freed African-American men received the vote while women did not. The American Equal Rights Association, which had formed in 1866 for the purpose of passing universal suffrage, divided in 1869 into the National Woman Suffrage Association (NWSA) led by Elizabeth Cady Stanton and Susan B. Anthony (1820–1906), and the American Woman Suffrage Association (AWSA) led by Henry Ward Beecher (1813–1887) and Lucy Stone (1818–1893). Stanton and Anthony rejected the secondary status of woman suffrage in the battle to gain universal suffrage and subsequently ended their affiliation with those reformers who accepted it. Beecher and Stone continued to work towards equal suffrage, but believed that the vote should first go to the freed male slaves and then, when abolitionists and other groups were ready, to women. In 1890, the campaign for woman suffrage unified as those two organizations merged and became the National American Woman Suffrage Association (NAWSA). Members of both organizations believed this unification marked a "new era in woman suffrage."[77]

Carrie Chapman Catt (1859–1947) succeeded Susan B. Anthony in 1900 as president of the new National American Woman Suffrage Association. Noted for her skills as an orator, Catt represented the NAWSA for four years throughout the country. She resigned from the presidency in 1904 because of her husband's ill health and an increasing interest in the international suffrage movement of the International Council of Women.[78]

Anna Howard Shaw (1847–1919), Anthony's close friend, served as next president of the NAWSA from 1900 to 1914. Shaw wrote that the dying Susan B. Anthony had asked Shaw to lead the suffrage campaign and remain NAWSA president for as long as she was "well enough to do the work."[79] Anthony forewarned Shaw of the "inevitable jealousies and misunderstandings" and the "criticism and misrepresentation" she would encounter as president.[80] Shaw kept her promise to Anthony and remained president for eleven years, during which time she energetically committed herself to woman suffrage. However, critics of Shaw's presidency charged that she lacked administrative skills, the ability to work with others, and above all, good judgement. Between 1904 and 1914, Shaw's opponents blamed her for NAWSA's lack of political direction or plans to promote a federal suffrage act.[81]

The woman suffrage movement experienced such diminished political activity during the late nineteenth and early twentieth century that historian Eleanor Flexner and contemporary suffragists described this period as the "doldrums." Anthony's death and Shaw's ineffective leadership confined NAWSA's efforts to a few local and state campaigns which offered no real chance for change in the status of women. In her book, *Jailed for Freedom* (1920), Doris Stevens wrote that after Anthony's death, "her followers had lost sight of her aggressive attack . . ." and the organization found itself "confined in a narrow circle of routine propaganda" which lacked "the power and initiative to extricate itself."[82]

However, activity among the NAWSA membership steadily rose in the two years following 1908 as its members obtained more than

404,000 names on a petition urging Congress to adopt a federal woman suffrage amendment. Flexner attributed further suffrage activity to Carrie Catt's involvement in the international woman suffrage movement, and to Harriet Stanton Blatch (1856–1940), daughter of Elizabeth Cady Stanton, who founded the Equality League of Self-Supporting Women in 1907. With the new members of the Equality League, which became the Women's Political Union in 1910, Blatch launched suffrage parades, open air meetings, and other proactive campaign strategies to convince New York legislators to support her cause.[83]

By 1913, militant suffragist Alice Paul (1885–1977) further shook the suffrage movement out of its doldrums as she revived Susan B. Anthony's "militant spirit" as chairman on the NAWSA Congressional Committee.[84] The day before Woodrow Wilson (1856–1924) took office as the twenty-eighth president of the United States in March 1913, Paul led a suffrage parade of 5,000 in Washington, D.C., to dramatize women's insistence on their political rights. Paul met President Wilson soon after he took office, accompanied by a deputation made up of suffragists Genevieve Stone, wife of an Illinois congressman, Mrs. Harvey W. Wiley, Ida Husted Harper (1851–1931), and Mary Bartlett Dixon, a registered nurse from Maryland. Paul questioned how Wilson's administration could "legislate for currency, tariff, and any other reform without first getting the consent of women to these reforms?"[85] This began the militant campaign led by Alice Paul and Lucy Burns (1879–1966) to convince the federal government of women's growing concern for political rights.[86]

Together, Burns, vice chairman of the NAWSA Congressional Committee, and Paul founded the Congressional Union for Woman Suffrage, with the support of NAWSA president Shaw, in April 1913.[87] Activists in the Congressional Union focused all their energy on passage of a federal suffrage amendment, and eventually severed their affiliation with the National American Woman Suffrage Association in 1914. Influenced by Paul's dynamic leadership, several smaller woman suffrage associations merged with the Congressional Union in 1917 and became the small but militant National Woman's Party (NWP). Following the British suffragist tactic of holding the party in power accountable, and despite United States' entry into World War I, this smaller suffrage organization refocused public attention on its work through suffrage parades, deputations to the president, petitions to congress, and arrests and imprisonment of members, subsequently earning them greater power and recognition than the larger, more conservative NAWSA. The NWP attracted a younger, college-educated membership who willingly faced courtroom appearances, endured forced feedings and months of illegal imprisonment to support successful passage of the federal woman suffrage amendment. Thus, Paul and the NWP escalated the activities within the woman suffrage movement in the second decade of the twentieth century.[88]

Although ideology and methodology espoused by suffrage supporters varied, as did their social, educational, and economic backgrounds, all suffragists shared the common goal of political equality for women. A large force within the ranks of suffragists was the American middle-class woman who had benefited from the increased educational opportunities available to women in the twentieth century. These women were more educated, politically astute, and more focused on the need for social reform than their nineteenth-century counterparts in the suffrage campaign. Predominantly middle-class nineteenth-century suffragists had always argued for suffrage because they saw it as their natural right and a means of protecting their homes and children. The "natural right" argument never fully disappeared from the suffragist rationale, but was replaced by the expediency argument which assumed that social reform in the twentieth century could only be achieved with the women's vote.[89]

The suffrage campaign between 1900 and 1920 was strongly influenced by the ideology of middle-class women and social feminism. For some middle-class women, just obtaining the vote was enough of a reason to support suffrage, while others felt that the vote would help them attain a particular desired political goal. However, working-class women were unswayed by middle-class arguments that the vote would give women political representation or would avail women of their natural rights as citizens or would allow them to protect their homes and children.[90]

Reform, rather than revolution, linked suffragists to other movements of the Progressive Era. Membership in the General Federation of Women's Clubs (1889), the Association of Collegiate Alumnae (1882), the Woman's Christian Temperance Union (1874), and other organizations brought together many reform-minded, middle-class, educated women who may also have been suffragists. Their commitment to woman suffrage varied within each organization and reflected a wide spectrum of ideas about women's rights.[91] The settlement house movement, organized into the National Federation of Settlements in 1911, attracted younger educated women from similar middle-class backgrounds determined to meet the social needs of lower and working class communities. Settlements in urban poor communities provided reformers with great opportunities for social housekeeping activities. Survival of the city and the health of its occupants relied on the reformers' ability to argue for playgrounds, labor laws, and well baby stations. Affluent members of settlement houses rallied behind working women who unionized, opposing unsafe working conditions and long hours of underpaid work. Settlement house reformers learned firsthand from working women about the miserable conditions they encountered daily in the factories, and thus the reformers were better able to agitate for political change. Lillian Wald, founder of Henry Street Settlement in New York City, described the impact when "fashionable women's clubs held meetings to hear the story from the lips of girl strikers themselves," and their resulting disapproval of the "judges who sentenced the young strikers to prison . . ." Many of the members of clubs and settlements, who "had never known the bitterness of poverty or oppression," marched in protest along side the striking women.[92]

During the late nineteenth and early twentieth centuries, several avenues to enact reforms existed for middle- and upper-class women interested in the plight of the working girl. The National Consumers' League (NCL) began in 1890 in New York City in response to a mass meeting of retail shop girls. By 1899, NCL had organized other leagues in cities throughout the country. Florence Kelley (1859–1932) became a prominent reform figure as a result of her activities as secretary of the NCL and her work with Jane Addams (1860–1935) at Hull House in Chicago and with Lillian Wald at Henry Street in New York.[93]

Another opportunity for middle- and upper-class women to join together in social reform existed in the National Women's Trade Union League (NWTUL), organized in 1903. Its motto, "The Eight-hour Day; A Living Wage; To Guard the Home"[94] brought together a unique membership of women whose religious, political, and economic backgrounds coexisted with the traditional middle-class reform ethic. Working women, Jewish women, and socialist women all found a home within the National Women's Trade Union. On behalf of the working women's activities in social reform Wald wrote that, "those who are familiar with factory and shop conditions are convinced that [only] through organization and not through the appeal to pity can permanent reforms be assured."[95] The success of the NWTUL relied on the support that women from varied social, economic, and political backgrounds gave to each other. Wald concluded that this gave ". . . practical expression to their belief that with them [women] and through them the realization of the ideals of democracy can be advanced."[96]

The fervor of social reform spawned associations which enabled women to claim their right to protest for change and improve the lives of all women. Working-class and middle-class women believed that woman suffrage would assure them political, social, and economic equality. Moreover, working-class women and middle-class women supported suffrage because they wanted to control their work. Thus, for most women of the progressive reform era, regardless of their economic class, interest in obtaining suffrage rested in their desire to control their lives. Similarly, for women in the newly emerging nursing profession, suffrage seemed as crucial to gaining and maintaining control of their professional lives.[97]

Late twentieth-century historian Ellen DuBois, who studied the political thought of Elizabeth Cady Stanton, theorized that a "woman's rights feminism"[98] had emerged in response to women's culture during the middle of the nineteenth century. As one of the original leaders in the suffrage movement, Stanton had vigorously opposed constraints that the nineteenth-century women's culture placed on all women. Stanton argued that political thought should replace the stifling nature of religious piety, self-development should replace the ideology of self-sacrifice, and woman's equal rights should replace the notion of woman's special and limited mission. Thus, Stanton challenged the validity and basis of nineteenth-century woman's sphere.[99]

In the late nineteenth and early twentieth century, a form of "nursing rights" feminism[100] developed that paralleled Stanton's political theory. Graduates of the late nineteenth-century nurse training schools organized professional nursing associations to gain control of nursing education and nursing practice. Their political battles focused on state registration of nurses, which designated who qualified as a registered nurse and defined the legal parameters of nursing practice. Trained nurses challenged previously held images of nursing derived from a woman's culture of unpaid self-sacrifice and unfailing religious obedience. Nursing leaders embraced a professional model that called for uniform standards for nursing education, rejected the image of the angel of mercy, stressed self-realization rather than self-sacrifice, demanded financial reward for services rendered, and worked for achieving women's equal status with men. In essence, nursing leaders worked for the emancipation of the nursing profession.[101]

Although another late twentieth-century historian, Barbara Melosh, wrote that most nursing leaders at the turn of the century did not identify their goals in terms of feminism, their commitment to the developing nursing profession and their efforts to claim professional privileges implicitly challenged and unsettled traditional and patriarchal constraints on women in the work force.[102] However, while nursing leaders worked for change, some nurses wrote in defense of the mission, religious calling, and moral tone of nursing. Thus, to some historians in the 1980s, a split between the leaders of the modern nursing movement and the more traditional practicing nurses seemed apparent by the first decade of the twentieth century.[103]

Between 1873 and 1920 many trained nurses came from the same middle-class background as the majority of suffrage supporters. However, whether trained nurses were among the leadership or within the rank and file, their arguments for suffrage paralleled those of both working- and middle-class women. Women suffragists appealed to the working class by arguing that the vote affected their ability to earn their livelihoods. Trained nurses echoed the middle-class argument which called for control of their political, social, and economic status, applying these arguments to the issues of their control of nursing education, nursing practice, and their ability to earn a living. Control of the profession hinged on liberating the political, social, and economic constraints placed on the growing nursing profession in the patriarchal society.[104] Additionally, nurses saw suffrage as a means of creating a healthier society and therefore wanted the vote to promote the changes needed for the greater good of society.

Soon after the establishment of the first nurse training schools in the late nineteenth century, nursing leaders had the foresight to harness the independent energy of newly trained nurses into an organizational force via nursing alumnae associations. Whether from a middle-class or a working-class background, the newly trained nurse represented the "new woman," one who was educated, financially independent, and seeking self-determination. Between 1873 and 1893, nurse training schools provided women a professional education, financial independence, and collegial relationships. Following 1873, new schools emerged and graduated new generations of trained nurses who contributed to the modern nursing movement and to the woman movement. The need to organize into professional associations became one of the driving forces within nursing by 1893. Thus, in keeping with activities of other women during the Progressive Era, nurses organized, worked for social reforms, and advocated control of the ballot. However, the professional nursing organizations were singular among contemporary women's associations because nursing advocates actively sought control of their professional destiny. Trained nurses and the emerging nursing profession contributed to and benefited from the woman's movement and the impending battle for woman suffrage.

NOTES

1. Louise Darche, "Proper Organization of Training Schools in America," in *Nursing of the Sick, 1893, Papers and Discussions from the International Congress of Charities, Correction, and Philanthropy,* ed. Isabel Hampton (New York: National League for Nursing Education, 1949), 93.

2. Angela Marie Howard Zophy, "For the Improvement of My Sex: Sarah Josepha Hale's Editorship of 'Godey's Lady's Book,' 1837–1877," Ph.D. diss., University of Ohio, 1978 (Ann Arbor, MI: University Microfilms International, order no. 7819687).

3. Eleanor Flexner, *Century of Struggle: The Woman's Rights Movement in the United States* (Cambridge, MA: Belknap Press of Harvard University Press, 1959), 62–70. This chapter explores the attitudes held by some of the organizers of the suffrage movement.

4. Susan Reverby, *Ordered to Care: The Dilemma of American Nursing, 1850–1945* (Cambridge: Cambridge University Press, 1987), 11–21.

5. Elizabeth Cady Staton, Susan B. Anthony, and Matilda Joslyn Gage, *History of Woman Suffrage,* 6 vols. (New York: Fowler & Wells, 1881–1922), I: 816, as quoted in Gerda Lerner, *The Female Experience:*

An American Documentary (Indianapolis: The Bobbs-Merrill Company, 1977), 417.

6. Nancy Cott, *The Bonds of Womanhood: "Woman's Sphere" in New England, 1780–1930* (New Haven: Yale University Press); Robert L. Daniels, *American Women in the 20th Century: The Festival of Life* (San Diego: Harcourt Brace Jovanovich, 1987), 4–9; Lerner, *Female Experience,* xxxi–xxxiii; Glenda Riley, *Inventing The American Woman: A Perspective on Women's History 1607–1877,* vol. 1 (Arlington Heights, IL: Harlan Davidson, 1986), 63–88; Sheila Rothman, *A Woman's Proper Place: A History of Changing Ideals and Practices, 1870 to the Present* (New York, Basic Books), 13–27, for discussion of woman's separate sphere; Phillip G. Hubert Jr., "The Trained Nurse," in *The Woman's Book,* vol. 1 (New York: Charles Scribner's Sons, 1894), 36–44; William King, *Woman: Her Position, Influence, and Achievement Throughout the Civilized World. Her Biography—Her History From the Garden of Eden to the Twentieth Century* (Springfield, MA: The King Richardson Co., 1903), 624–625; Zophy, "Hale's Editorship," for references to Sarah Josepha Hale's promotion of a woman's separate sphere.

7. Rothman, *Woman's Proper Place,* 21–26, for discussion of the attributes of the nineteenth-century virtuous women.

8. Cott, *The Bonds of Womanhood,* 62.

9. Riley, *Inventing the American Woman,* I:5–8.

10. Cott, *The Bonds of Womanhood,* 105.

11. Barbara Miller Solomon, *In the Company of Educated Women,* (New Haven, CT: Yale University Press, 1985), 50–61; Nicholas C. Burckel, "Oberlin College," in *Handbook of American Women's History,* eds. Angela Howard Zophy and Frances M. Kavenik (Garland Reference Library of the Humanities V. 696, 1990), 445. For history and discussion of coeducation in America, see chapter reference notes 14, 15, and 19.

12. Cott, *Bonds of Womanhood,* 101–125; Frederick Randolph, "Emma Hart Willard," in *Notable American Women 1607–1950: A Biographical Dictionary,* vol. 3, eds. Edward T. James, Janet Wilson James, and Paul S. Boyer (Cambridge, MA: The Belknap Press of Harvard University Press, 1971), 610–613; see John Lord, *The Life of Emma Willard* (New York: Appleton, 1873) and Alma Lutz, *Emma Willard: Daughter of Democracy* (Boston: Houghton Mifflin, 1929) for biographies on Willard; Solomon, *Educated Women,* 14–26; Robert G. Waite, "Emma Hart Willard," in Zophy and Kavenik, *Handbook,* 662–3.

13. Barbara M. Cross, "Catherine Esther Beecher," in *NAW,* I: 121–124; Cott, *Bonds of Womanhood,* 101–125; Kathryn Kish Sklar, *Catherine*

Beecher: A Study in American Domesticity (New Haven, Yale University Press, 1973), 59–77; Solomon, *Educated Women,* 14–26.

14. Cott, *Bonds of Womanhood,* 101–125; Helen Lefkowitz Horowitz, *Alma Mater: Design and Experience in the Women's Colleges from Their Nineteenth-Century Beginnings to the 1930s* (New York: Alfred A. Knopf, 1984), 9–27; Sydney R. MacLean, "Zilpah Polly Grant" and "Mary Lyon" in *NAW,* II: 73–75, and II: 443–447; Sklar, *Beecher,* 59–77; Solomon, *Educated Women,* 14–26.

15. Elizabeth A. Daniels, *Matthew Vassar 1792–1868: More Than a Brewer* (Poughkeepsie, NY: Vassar College, 1992), 5–14, for a biographical essay of Matthew Vassar; Horowitz, *Alma Mater,* 28–41; for Hale's influence on Vassar and other women's schools, see Zophy, *Hale's Editorship,* 111–129.

16. Horowitz, *Alma Mater,* 42–45 for a full discussion of the architectural design and comparison of Wellesley to Mt. Holyoke and Vassar; Margaret E. Taylor, "The Founders and the Early Presidents," in *Wellesley College 1875–1975: A Century of Women,* ed. Jean Glasscock (Wellesley, MA: Wellesley College, 1975), 1–23.

17. See summary of coeducational schools and their performance to 1875 on p. 18.

18. Reverend L. Clark Seelye, *The Need of a Collegiate Education for Woman* (Massachusetts, American Institute of Instruction at North Adams, 1874), 25.

19. Horowitz, *Alma Mater,* 80.

20. Elizabeth Deering Hanscom, *Sophia Smith and the Beginnings of Smith College* (Northampton, MA: Smith College, 1926), for biographical history of Smith and Smith College; Seelye, *Collegiate Education,* 5–35, for arguments favoring single-sex colleges; see Margaret Storrs Grierson, "Sophia Smith" in *NAW,* III: 318–320; Horowitz, *Alma Mater,* 69–81; Harriet C. Seelye, "Festivals in American Colleges For Women: At Smith," *The Century Magazine,* 49 no. 3 (January 1895): 432–437 for description of student celebrations and student life; Bonnie Smith, "Smith College," in Zophy and Kavenik, *Handbook,* 554–555.

21. Edith Finch, *Carey Thomas of Bryn Mawr* (New York: Harper & Brothers, 1947), 132–160 for description of the opening of Bryn Mawr and 246–257 for discussion of Carey's involvement in woman suffrage organizations; Rita Rubinstein Heller, "Bryn Mawr Summer School for Women Workers," in Zophy and Kavenik, *Handbook,* 96; Horowitz, *Alma Mater,* 105–142; Lawrence R. Veysey, "Martha Carey Thomas," in *NAW,* 3: 446–450.

22. Annette Baxter, "Ella Weed," in *NAW,* 3:556–557; Henry Steele Commager, "Mary Elizabeth Mapes Dodge," in *NAW,* 1:495–496; Horowitz, *Alma Mater,* 134–142; Linda Kerber, "Annie Nathan Meyer," in *Notable American Women, The Modern Period; A Biographical Dictionary,* eds. Barbara Sicherman and Carol Hurd Green (Cambridge, MA: The Belknap Press of Harvard University Press, 1980), 473–474; Alice Duer Miller and Susan Myers, *Barnard College; The First Fifty Years* (New York: Columbia University Press, 1939), 3–34.

23. Horowitz, *Alma Mater,* 95–104; Solomon, *Educated Women,* 55; John L. Rury, "Radcliffe College," in Zophy and Kavenik, *Handbook,* 503–4.

24. Riley, *Inventing The American Woman,* I: 88–95; Solomon, *Educated Women,* 14–26, 27–61, for further readings about women and education in the nineteenth century; see Rothman, *Woman's Proper Place,* 26–42, regarding the attempt to counteract the accusations that education for a woman was hazardous to her health.

25. Zophy, *Hale's Editorship,* 111–129, for full discussion of Sarah Josepha Hale's role in promoting women's education. Hale and her conservative colleagues deemed women superior to men and eschewed politics as too vulgar for women.

26. Daniel Scott Smith, "Family Limitation, Social Control, and Domestic Feminism in Victorian America," in *A Heritage of Her Own: Toward a New Social History of American Women,* eds. Nancy F. Cott and Elizabeth H. Pleck (New York: Touchstone/Simon and Schuster, 1979), 222–45; Angela Howard Zophy, "Domestic Feminism," in Zophy and Kavenik, *Handbook,* 163–164.

27. Sir Edward Cook, *The Life of Florence Nightingale,* vol. 1 (London: Macmillan and Co., 1913), 439–455, for discussion of Nightingale as the founder of the modern nursing movement; see Lavinia Dock, "Some Urgent Social Claims," *AJN* (July 1907): 896, for Dock's assessment that the modern nursing movement was an outcome of the woman movement; see Florence Nightingale, *Notes on Nursing: What It Is, and What It Is Not* (1860; reprint, New York: Dover Publications, 1969), 7–140, to understand Nightingale's opinion that pure air, nutritious food, adequate lighting, and proper ventilation contributed to decreased morbidity rates and enhanced the curative process.

28. Nightingale, *Notes on Nursing,* 10–11.

29. Ibid., 9.

30. Cook, *Nightingale,* 1:445; also see Vern Bullough, Bonnie Bullough, and Marietta Stanton, eds., *Florence Nightingale and Her Era: A Collection of New Scholarship* (New York: Garland Publishing Company,

1990), for readings of Nightingale's influence on the modern nursing movement.

31. Susan Reverby, "The Search for the Hospital Yardstick: Nursing and the Rationalization of Hospital Work," in *Sickness and Health in America: Readings in the History of Medicine and Public Health,* 2nd ed., eds. Judith Walzer Leavitt and Ronald L. Numbers (Madison, WI: University of Wisconsin Press, 1985), 206–216, for recognition of nursing's influential role in changing hospital care in America following implementation of Nightingale's reforms.

32. Paul Starr, *The Social Transformation of American Medicine* (New York: Basic Books, 1982), 145–179; Morris J. Vogel, "The Transformation of the American Hospital, 1850–1920" in *Health Care in America: Essays in Social History,* eds. Susan Reverby and David Rosner (Philadelphia: Temple University Press, 1979), 105–116; Charles E. Rosenberg, *The Care of Strangers: The Rise of America's Hospital System* (New York: Basic Books Inc., 1987), 212–236, for a discussion of the changes in American hospitals between 1850 and 1920.

33. Bonnie Bullough and Vern Bullough, "The Origins of Modern American Nursing: The Civil War Era," *Nursing Forum* 2 (1963): 13–27, for discussion of nursing care in hospitals prior to the opening of nurse training schools in 1873; Reverby, "Hospital Yardstick," in Leavitt and Numbers, *Sickness and Health,* 206; Rosenberg, *The Care of Strangers,* 213.

34. Josephine Dolan, *Nursing in Society: A Historical Perspective* 13th ed. (Philadelphia: W.B. Saunders, 1973), 159–160; Charles Dickens, *The Life and Adventures of Martin Chuzzlewit* (Chicago: Belford, Clarke and Company, n.d.), [published in 1844]. Dickens portrayed untrained nursing care prior to the Nightingale reforms.

35. Bullough and Bullough, "The Civil War Era," 13–27; Lerner, *Female Experience,* 150, 180–182; Inez Haynes Irwin, *Angels and Amazons: A Hundred Years of American Women* (Garden City, NY: Doubleday, Doran & Company, 1933), 146–156; Roberta Tierney, "The Beneficent Revolution: Hospital Nursing during the Civil War," Bullough, Bullough, and Stanton, *Nightingale and Her Era,* 138–149; Reverby, *Ordered to Care,* 11–21, for discussion of a woman's duty to nurse.

36. Lavinia L. Dock and Isabel Maitland Stewart, *A Short History of Nursing from the Earliest Times to the Present Day* (New York: G.P. Putnam's Sons, 1931), 148–150, for discussion of nursing during the Civil War; Roberta Tierney, "The Beneficent Revolution: Hospital Nursing During the Civil War" in Bullough, Bullough, and Stanton, *Nightingale and*

Her Era, 138–151; Frank Moore, *Women of the War; Their Heroism and Self-Sacrifice* (Hartford, CT: S.S. Scranton Co., 1866), for accounts of volunteer nurses during the Civil War.

37. Moore, *Women of the War,* 571–77, for a description of the Sanitary Commission; Robert D. Cross, "Louisa Lee Schuyler," in *NAW,* 3: 244–46; Vern Bullough, "Louisa Lee Schuyler," Vern L. Bullough, Olga Maranjian Church, and Alice P. Stein, *American Nursing: A Biographical Dictionary,* vol. 1 (New York: Garland Publishing Company, 1988), 284–85; Elizabeth H. Thompson, "Elizabeth Blackwell," *NAW,* 1: 161–65; and A. Gretchen McNeely and Irene Palmer, "Elizabeth Blackwell," Bullough, Bullough, and Stein, *American Nursing,* II: 30–3; Cook, *Nightingale* II: 8–10; and Dock and Stewart, *Short History,* 128–29.

38. Moore, *Women of the War,* 592–3; Rosenberg, *The Care of Strangers,* 97–99.

39. Irwin, *Angels and Amazons,* 146–162, for effect the Civil War had on nursing education; Dock and Stewart, *Short History,* 150–52; Isabel Maitland Stewart, *The Education of Nurses: Historical Foundations and Modern Trends* (New York: Macmillan Company, 1948), 84.

40. Cook, *Nightingale* 1:456–467; Janice Cooke Feigenbaum, "Students Wanted: Women Need Not Apply: A Historical Review of Ideas on Women's Place in Higher Education During the Nightingale Era," in Bullough, Bullough, and Stanton, *Nightingale and Her Era,* 188–205.

41. Cook, *Nightingale,* I: 467; see Stewart, *Education of Nurses,* 84–87, for recommendations brought before the American Medical Association by Dr. Samuel D. Gross, professor of surgery at Jefferson Medical College in Philadelphia, in an attempt to improve Nightingale's plan by placing nursing education under the control of the medical profession.

42. Editorial Comment, "Progress and Reaction," *AJN,* 8 (February 1908): 333–334.

43. Cook, *Nightingale,* 1:441, "'There is an old legend,'" wrote Miss Nightingale at the beginning of her pamphlet on Kaiserswerth, "that the nineteenth century is to be the 'century of women.'" See Florence Nightingale, *Cassandra,* in R. Strachey, *"The Cause": A Short History of the Women's Movement in Great Britain* (London: G. Bell and Sons, 1928), for Nightingale's 1852 feminist essay, *Cassandra,* that reflected some of her feminist views; Peggy Chinn, "What's in a Name???," in *Re-membering Our Heritage: Cassandra Radical Feminist Network* (no publishing information); Elaine Showalter, "Florence Nightingale's Feminist Complaint: Women, Religion, and Suggestions for Thought," *Signs* (Spring 1981): 395–412.

44. Cook, *Nightingale* 1:465, for brief description of a Nightingale-trained nurse in America: Alice Fisher (1839–1888), regenerated the Blockey Hospital in Philadelphia; see Sharon Murphy, "Alice Fisher," Bullough, Sentz, and Stein, *American Nursing*, 2: 113–16; *see* "Map Showing Widespread Influence of the Nightingale System of Nursing Education During the First 50 Years, 1860–1910," in Dock and Stewart, *Short History*, 189.

45. Stewart, *Education of Nurses*, 84.

46. Lena Dixon Dietz and Aurelia R. Lehozky, *History and Modern Nursing*, 2nd ed. (Philadelphia: F. A. Davis Co., 1967), 95; Dock and Stewart, *Short History*, 146–52; Phillip Kalisch and Beatrice Kalisch, *The Advance of American Nursing*, 2nd ed. (Boston: Little, Brown & Company, 1986), 88–89.

47. Dietz and Lehozky, *Modern Nursing*, 94–103; Dock and Stewart, *Short History*, 146–52; Kalisch and Kalisch, *Advances*, 100–104; Linda Richards, *Reminiscences of Linda Richards*, 2nd ed. (Boston: Whitcomb & Barrows, 1915).

48. Dock and Stewart, *Short History*, 155.

49. May Ayres Burgess, *Nurses, Patients, and Pocketbooks* (New York: Committee on the Grading of Nursing Schools, 1928), 34–35; Dock and Stewart, *Short History*, 155–56; Dietz and Lehozky, *Modern Nursing*, 97–9; Kalisch and Kalisch, *Advances*, 71–106.

50. Dock and Stewart, *Short History*, 154.

51. Franklin H. North, "A New Profession For Women," *The Century Illustrated Monthly Magazine*, 25 no.1 (November 1882): 39; and the Alumnae Association of Bellevue School of Nursing, *The Alumnae Association of the Bellevue School of Nursing* (New York: The Alumnae Association of the Bellevue School of Nursing, 1989), 12–24, for a photocopy of Nightingale's letter. The presence of the original letter in the Bellevue archives is difficult to ascertain because there is some confusion by hospital archivists as to where Bellevue's records have been kept since its centennial celebration.

52. See Alumnae Association of Bellevue School of Nursing, *The Alumnae Association of the Bellevue School of Nursing*, 25, for the goals of the training school for nurses.

53. Stewart, *Education of Nurses*, 47.

54. Ibid., 78.

55. Ibid., 53.

56. Isabel Hampton Robb, "The Past, Present, and Future of Nursing in the United States of America," *AJN*, 11 (October 1910): 25–26; Stewart, *Education of Nurses*, 90–91.

57. Stewart, *Education of Nurses*, 98.

58. Lucy Ridgely Seymer, *A General History of Nursing* (New York, The Macmillan Co., 1933), 166; Stewart, *Education of Nurses*, 154–156.

59. Stewart, *Education of Nurses*, 166; Stewart explained that this "change in terminology . . . is worth noting because 'pupil' implies intellectual immaturity and guardianship while 'student' is used to describe more mature, independent, self-directing learners."

60. Ibid., 99–101.

61. Louise Darche in Stewart, *Education of Nurses*, 104; Louise Darche, "Proper Organization of Training Schools in America," in Part III, "Nursing of the Sick," *Hospitals, Dispensaries and Nursing: Papers and Discussions in the International Congress of Charities, Correction, and Philanthropy, Section III, Chicago, June 12–17th, 1893*, eds. Johns S. Billings and Henry M. Hurd (Baltimore: Johns Hopkins Press, 1984), 516–517.

62. May Ayres Burgess, "How Fast Has Nursing Grown," *Nurses, Patients, and Pocketbooks* (New York: Committee on the Grading of Nursing Schools, 1928), 33–47; Dock and Stewart, *Short History*, 160; Adelaide Nutting, "Some Problems of Training Schools For Nurses," in *A Sound Economic Basis For Schools of Nursing and Other Addresses*, ed. Adelaide Nutting (1925; reprint, New York: Garland Publishing Company, 1984), 34.

63. Burgess, *Nurses, Patients, and Pocketbooks*, 37, 40.

64. Nettie Birnbach, "The Genesis of the Nurse Registration Movement in the United States, 1893–1903," Ed.D. diss., Teachers College, Columbia University, 1982 (*Dissertation Abstracts International, 44,* 455B); Susan Reverby, "A Caring Dilemma: Womanhood and Nursing in Historical Perspective," *Nursing Research,* 36 no. 1 (January/February 1987): 8.

65. Burgess, *Nurses, Patients, and Pocketbooks,* 18, 28; The Committee on the Grading of Nursing Schools compiled statistical information to acertain the supply and demand for nursing services, the kind of information nurses needed to know, how to teach nurses this information, and the evaluation of schools of nursing. Twenty-one members sat on the committee, fourteen appointed from different national organizations (i.e., the NLNE, the ANA, the NOPHN, the American Medical Association), and seven elected to serve as members at large. The committee worked on this project for five years, funded at first by a donation from

Mrs. Chester Bolton, a member of the committee, and later by the Rockefeller Foundation, the Commonwealth Fund, and nurses.

66. Nightingale, *Notes on Nursing,* 135.

67. Ibid.

68. Ibid., 135–6; Smith, "Family Limitation, Social Control, and Domestic Feminism in Victorian America," in *A Heritage of Her Own,* 238–40; Angela Howard Zophy, "Domestic Feminism," in Zophy and Kavenik, *Handbook,* 163–164.

69. Lillian Wald, "Work of Women in Municipal Affairs," *Proceedings of the Sixth Annual Convention of the National League for Nursing Education* (Harrisburg, PA: Harrisburg Publishing, 1900), 54–57; speech is reprinted in Susan Reverby, ed., *Annual Conventions 1893–1899 ASSTSN* (New York: Garland Publishing Company, 1985), 54–57, and Nettie Birnbach and Sandra Lewenson, *First Words: Selected Addresses from the National League for Nursing 1894–1933* (New York: National League of Nursing Press, 1991), 315–318.

70. Daniel, *American Women in the 20th Century,* 33–35; Zophy, "Social Feminism," and "Social Housekeeping," in Zophy and Kavenik, *Handbook,* 557, 558; Mary I. Wood, *The History of the General Federation of Women's Clubs,* (New York: General Federation of Women's Clubs, 1912), 22–40.

71. Lavinia L. Dock, "The Duty of the Society in Public Work," *Proceedings of the Tenth Annual Convention of the ASSTSN* (Baltimore: J.H. Furst, 1904), 77–79; reprinted in Birnbach and Lewenson, *First Words,* 319–321; and Wald, "Work of Women in Municipal Affairs," 54–57.

72. Mary B. Dixon, "Votes for Women," *Nurses' Journal of the Pacific Coast,* 4 (October 1908): 442.

73. Bullough and Bullough, "The Origins of Modern American Nursing: The Civil War Era," 14, for nursing as an outgrowth of the woman's rights movement; and Sandra Lewenson, *The Relationship Among the Four Professional Nursing Organizations and Woman Suffrage: 1893–1920,* Ed.D. diss., Teachers College, Columbia University, 1989, Ann Arbor, MI, University Microfilms International, order no. 9002561), 1–17.

74. Report of the Woman's Rights Convention, (reprint, Easter National Park and Monuments Association), 7.

75. The following sources provided the background material used in this section: Eleanor Flexner, *Century of Struggle: The Woman's Rights Movement in the United States,* rev. ed. (Cambridge, MA: Belknap Press of Harvard University Press, 1959, 1975), vii–xiii; Irwin, *Angels and*

Amazons, 238–266; Aileen Kraditor, *The Ideas of the Woman Suffrage Movement 1890–1920* (Garden City, NY: Anchor Books-Doubleday, 1971), 1–63; readings from Aileen Kraditor, ed., *Up From the Pedestal: Selected Writings in the History of American Feminism* (Chicago: Quadrangle Books, 1970) 183–287; David Morgan, "Woman Suffrage in Britain and America in the Early Twentieth Century," in *Contrast and Connection: Bicentennial Essays in Anglo-American History,* eds. H.C. Allen and Roger Thompson (Athens, OH: Ohio University Press, 1976), 272–295; William L. O'Neil, *Everyone was Brave: The Rise and Fall of Feminism in America* (Chicago: Quadrangle Books, 1969), 49–76; Andrew Sinclair, *The Emancipation of the American Woman,* [originally published in hardcover under the title, *The Better Half*] (New York: Harper Colophon Books, 1965), 144–150.

76. Ellen Carol DuBois, *Feminism and Suffrage: The Emergence of an Independent Women's Movement in America 1848–1869* (Ithaca, NY: Cornell University Press, 1978), 21–55; Flexner, *Century of Struggle,* 90–91; Gaylè J. Hardy, "Sojourner Truth," in *American Nursing: A Biographical Dictionary,* vol. 2, eds. Vern L. Bullough, Lilli Sentz, and Alice P. Stein (New York: Garland Publishing Company, 1992), 330–2; Irwin, *Angels and Amazons,* 100–01 for text of Truth's speech delivered in Akron, Ohio, in 1851; Saunders Redding, "Sojourner Truth," in *Notable American Women* 3:479–481; Barbara Mayer Wertheimer, *We Were There: The Story of Working Women in America* (New York: Pantheon Books, 1977), 138–143.

77. Kraditor, *Ideas,* 3; and DuBois, *Feminism and Suffrage,* 53–78.

78. Flexner, *Century of Struggle,* 243–47, for description of Carrie Catt and Anna Howard Shaw; Eleanor Flexner, "Carrie Clinton Lane Chapman Catt," *Notable American Women,* I:309–13; Ellen Carol DuBois ed., *Elizabeth Cady Stanton–Susan B. Anthony Correspondence: Writings, Speeches* (New York: Schocken Books, 1981), 88–94, 178–182, for discussion of the split between suffragists and the merger of both groups in 1890, respectively.

79. Anna Howard Shaw, *The Story of a Pioneer* (New York: Harper & Brothers, 1915), 230.

80. Ibid., 232.

81. Flexner, "Anna Howard Shaw," *NAW,* III: 274–77; and Shaw, *Pioneer,* 234–5, for Shaw's account of her friendship with Anthony.

82. Doris Stevens, *Jailed for Freedom* (New York: Boni and Liveright, 1920), 8.

83. Flexner, *Century of Struggle,* 256; and Flexner, "Harriot Eaton Stanton Blatch," *NAW,* I: 172–174.

84. Stevens, *Jailed for Freedom,* 9.

85. Ibid., 23.

86. Flexner, *Century of Struggle,* 270–273.

87. Ibid., 274.

88. Cott, *Modern Feminism,* 53–81; Flexner, *Century of Struggle,* 274–5, [the Congressional Union severed its loosely affiliated status with National American Woman Suffrage Association in 1914]; Kraditor, *Ideas,* 1–11, 185–209; Stevens, *Jailed for Freedom,* 9, 21–60, for account of Alice Paul's work as suffrage organizer and for descriptions of terrorist treatment of imprisoned suffragist protesters; see Saundra K. Yelton, Neil W. Hogan and Angela Howard Zophy, "The National Woman's Party," and Ted C. Harris, "Alice Paul," in Zophy and Kavenik *Handbook,* 416–19 and 462–3, respectively.

89. Cott, *Modern Feminism,* 29–30; Flexner, *Century of Struggle* (rev. ed.), (257–270); Kraditor, *Ideas,* 39; and Kraditor, "The 'Expediency' Argument. II: Other Forms," in *Up From the Pedestal,* 266–287.

90. Kraditor, "The 'Expediency' Argument," 265–287.

91. O'Neil, *Everyone Was Brave,* 77–106.

92. Lillian Wald, *The House of Henry Street,* (New York: Henry Holt and Company 1915), 210.

93. O'Neil, *Everyone Was Brave,* 95–98; Louise Wade, "Florence Kelley," *NAW,* II: 316–319.

94. Wald, *The House on Henry Street,* 207.

95. Ibid., 207; O'Neil, *Everyone Was Brave,* 101.

96. Wald, *The House on Henry Street,* 207–8.

97. See Irwin, *Angels and Amazons,* Appendix, for description of women's organizations formed in the late nineteenth and early twentieth centuries, 443–499; O'Neil, *Everyone Was Brave,* 77–106, for a comparative history of many of the major women's associations at the turn of the twentieth century.

98. Ellen Carol DuBois, "Politics and Culture in Women's History: A Symposium," *Feminist Studies,* 6 no. 1 (Spring 1980): 30.

99. DuBois, "Politics and Culture," 28–36; and Dubois, *Stanton-Anthony,* 182–193; Elizabeth Cady Stanton, "The Solitude of Self," [Document 20, January 18, 1892] in Dubois, *Stanton-Anthony,* 246–54. In this 1890 address to the NAWSA, Stanton argued that granting women the vote was a matter of practical politics rather than gender, and that women as individual beings needed to be educated to become self-sufficient—

economically, politically, and emotionally. See Elizabeth Cady Stanton, *Eighty Years and More Reminiscences 1815–1897* (New York: Schocken Books, 1971), for development of Stanton's ideas.

100. "Nursing rights" is a term this author uses to describe the struggle of women in nursing to establish professional autonomy within the health care system.

101. Ethel Bedford Fenwick, "The International Council of Nurses, A Message From its President," *AJN*, 1 no. 11 (August 1901): 789, Fenwick hoped that international nursing councils would work for "graduate suffrage," as a means of obtaining needed nursing registration; A Character Sketch By An Intimate, "Foreign Delegates and Organization, Ethel Gordon Fenwick," 865, states "She [Fenwick] has proposed a simple basis—professional enfranchisement through State registration and self-government."

102. Barbara Melosh, *"The Physician's Hand": Work Culture and Conflict in American Nursing* (Philadelphia: Temple University Press, 1982), 22–29, 95, for discussion of professional ideology of nursing leaders and the traditional ideology of the nurse.

103. Ibid., 22; Reverby, *Ordered to Care*, 6.

104. Jo Ann Ashley, *Hospitals, Paternalism, and the Role of the Nurse,* (New York: Teachers College Press, 1976), 1–134. Throughout the book, Ashley argues the effects of paternalism on the development of the modern nursing movement in America.

2

Emancipation Through Organization

Organization is the power of the day. Without it nothing great is accomplished.

Sophia Palmer, 1897[1]

BETWEEN 1873 AND 1920, the newly trained graduate nurse replaced the unskilled nurse as hospitals and nurse training schools proliferated. Innovative in their approach to health care, pioneers of the new profession pushed forward the frontiers of nursing education and practice at these new schools and hospitals. Faced with opposition from hospital boards and medical doctors who wanted to control nurse training, these women had to be a "strong, determined, and intrepid set of workers . . . ." Like other social reformers of that time, they fought ". . . against physical dirt, disorder, . . . irresponsibility, political corruption, and every form of opposition and hostility."[2]

Even when hospitals seemingly supported their cause by establishing nurse training schools, nursing advocates had to struggle to assure that improved education and practice were the goals of the institution. Savvy hospital boards recognized the financial advantages a nurse training school brought to their institutions. Rather than hire graduate nurses who would have to be paid, hospitals could use nursing students to provide nursing care. Although in 1883 many hospitals paid training school students a stipend of anywhere from $9.00 a month up to $16.00 a month, depending on whether they were first- or second-year students, graduate nurses were paid from $25.00 up to $30.00 a month.[3] As a result, hospital boards primarily saw nurse training schools as an expedient means of securing a cheap source of specialized labor, thus relegating the educational purpose of nurse training to a secondary position.[4] Concerned about the educational misuse of students by some hospital schools, Louise Darche (1852–1899), an 1885 Bellevue Training School graduate and one of the founding members of the American Society of Superintendents of Training Schools for Nurses, warned potential nursing students in the nineteenth-century periodical, *The Delineator.* Darche wrote that so many hospitals "had been started with a view to providing a system of cheap nursing for small hospitals" and paid little attention to the needs of the nurse in training. Those interested in the profession should carefully look for an appropriate school, one that was connected with a larger hospital and could "supply a sufficient number and variety of cases to offer ample opportunity for practically observing and noting the signs and circumstances of different diseases." Rather than hastily enter a smaller school, she advised women to wait for an opening in one of the better training schools.[5] The early pioneers of nursing education continually experienced tension between a student's duty to the hospital and a student's need for education. Since hospitals with nurse training schools did not hire graduate nurses except for superintendent or head nurse positions, most new graduates worked outside the hospital as private duty nurses.[6] While enrolled in nurse training, students worked twelve-hour shifts on hospital wards and had little time off for recreation, relaxation, or study. Hospitals provided them with room, board and a small stipend. The quality of nursing care administered depended greatly on the hospital training school that the nurse attended. Each nurse training school decided its own entrance requirements and professional curriculum. The financial needs of the hospital, in most instances, dictated the candidates' qualifications and the type of education they received. Members of hospital boards and physicians often believed that if nurses were too educated, their ability to "nurse" would be jeopardized. They maintained the paternalistic stance that nurses did not need scientific knowledge to do the work they always did, ". . . that the old nurses were good enough . . . that the new nurses would be overtaught."[7] One physician wrote that "any intelligent, not necessarily educated woman can in short time acquire the skill to carry out with implicit obedience the physician's direction."[8] These men wanted nurses in hospitals to conform to a woman's role of subordination as perpetuated within the woman's sphere of domesticity. Thus, nursing pioneers struggled for a professional education, encountering opposition from those who wished nurses to maintain women's separate and secondary role in society.[9]

After a one- or two-year program at a hospital nurse training school, students graduated as trained nurses.[10] They found few jobs in hospitals following graduation, so most worked as private duty nurses providing nursing care for patients in their homes. Prior to the modern nurse movement, female family members and untrained attendants provided care to the sick at home under the supervision of young medical men. Once trained, nurses became private duty nurses for families in the home. However, the men lost some of the cases and their fees. According to pioneer nursing leaders and historians Lavinia Dock (1858–1956) and Isabel Stewart (1878–1963), this income loss generated some of the medical establishment's opposition to the modern nursing movement.[11]

Working alone on a case, private duty nurses became isolated from other nurses and felt that they needed to establish contact with colleagues from their former training schools. Newly formed alumnae associations provided graduates of nurse training schools with club life and a means of regaining the companionship they had once experienced while in training. These associations paralleled the developments of similar groups within other women's professions and of study groups among middle-class matrons who had attended institutions of higher education.[12]

One such group was the Association of Collegiate Alumnae (later known as the American Association of University Women), founded in 1882. The Association of Collegiate Alumnae returned college educated women to the yearned-for collegial relationships they shared during their college life. Once graduated from college, they found their intellectual lives barren, with few opportunities for social or economic advancement other than teaching. These women formed the Association of Collegiate Alumnae to support each other as they progressed from the private to the more public sphere of economic self-support and social reform. In addition to the collegiate alumnae, the late nineteenth- and early twentieth-century social reformers, involved in movements of social housekeeping and social feminism, formed groups which enabled women to collectively and publicly express themselves. Women in their various organizations earned a collective voice in America as progressive reforms emerged. The young profession of nursing could not help but be influenced by the national and international movement to organize.[13]

The profession of nursing, similarly engaged in developing women's intellect, self-supporting opportunities, and social reforms through nurse training schools, organized nursing associations in order to cultivate their collective voice. In 1888, one of the first nurse alumnae associations in America was established at the Training School for Nurses at the Woman's Hospital in Philadelphia. A year later, graduates from Bellevue Training School for Nurses in New York City organized an alumnae association. Bellevue graduates envisioned an alumnae association as a means of promoting fellowship among their graduates and as a means of financially supporting both their alma mater and other graduate nurses when needed. Illinois Training School graduates in Chicago organized an alumnae association in 1891, and graduates from the Johns Hopkins school in Baltimore organized one in 1892. Nursing superintendent Lystra Gretter (1858–1951), at the Farrand Training School at Harper Hospital in Detroit, assisted her school alumnae as they formed Michigan's first nursing association in 1893. Nurses from Massachusetts General Hospital in Boston organized in 1895, as did nurses from the Boston City Hospital a year later.[14] Alumnae associations linked nurses with their old training schools and their former classmates.

The scattered alumnae associations provided the basis from which the national associations could form and protect the interests of the graduate nurse on a more global scale. The first two national associations which formed prior to 1900 were the American Society of Superintendents of Training Schools for Nurses (hereafter called the Superintendents' Society) in 1893, and the Nurses' Associated Alumnae Association (hereafter called the Associated Alumnae) in 1896. The American Federation of Nurses (AFN) occupied a brief period in nursing history, lasting from 1900 until 1912,[15] and representing American nurses at meetings of the International Council of Women (ICW), and the National Council of Women (NCW). Two other national professional associations formed following 1900 focused on interests of special groups. African-American nurses formed the National Association of Colored Graduate Nurses (NACGN) in 1908 to address the problems they experienced as nurses and as black women. Public health nurses formed the National Organization for Public Health

Nurses (NOPHN) in 1912 to address the special needs of the newly emerging health care setting of public health and public health nursing.

Superintendents of nurse training schools and other nursing leaders between 1873 and 1893 entertained the ideas of association, affiliation, and organization.[16] Themselves graduates of the early nurse training schools, these professionals saw their educational freedom hampered by the attempts of those outside of nursing, such as hospital boards and physicians, to control nursing education. Therefore, they sought support from their colleagues as they defined and implemented educational reforms in nursing. Many nurses were responsible for this movement towards self-organization. Each of the national associations had its own leaders; however, many of these leaders and members actively participated in more than one nursing association. The following brief biographical sketches of some of nursing's leaders are chronologically organized by when an association was formed and by the multiple ties each nurse maintained.

Linda Richards (1841–1930), distinguished as the first graduate nurse in America following completion of a one-year nurse training course given at the New England Hospital for Women and Children in Boston in 1873, worked actively in the growth of nurse training at the Bellevue Training School in New York and at the Boston Training School in Boston. Recognized for her pioneer role in nursing, her peers elected her the first president of the Superintendents' Society in 1894.[17]

Isabel Hampton Robb (1860–1910), one of the founders of the Superintendents' Society and the Associated Alumnae, graduated from nurse training in 1883 after completing a two-year course at Bellevue Hospital in New York. From then on, Robb moved into leadership positions throughout her short-lived career. She worked as the superintendent of nurses at the Illinois Training School for Nurses at Cook County Hospital in Chicago and later as superintendent of nurses at the Johns Hopkins nurse training school, which opened in 1889. In 1893, Robb presented a paper regarding the importance of forming a national association for graduate nurses to the International Congress of Charities, Correction, and Philanthropy held in Chicago during the Columbian Exposition. Robb had been chair of the nursing subdivision at the international congress at the exposition and became one of the founders of the Superintendents' Society formed as a result of the international meeting. The Superintendents' Society was followed by the formation of the Associated Alumnae (to be discussed later in this chapter), and Robb was elected its first president in 1897. She also helped to establish the post-graduate course in hospital economics for nurses at Teachers College, Columbia University in New York. Among her many organizational activities, Robb helped initiate the Associated Alumnae official journal, *The American Journal of Nursing,* in 1900. As an invited member of the International Council of Women in 1899, Robb participated in the newly formed International Council of Nurses. Lavinia Dock (1858–1956) described Robb as one of nursing's "determinedly feminist" leaders, remembering "the close affinity between Miss Hampton and the Baltimore leaders of feminism . . . ."[18] Hampton proved by her actions to be feministic in her political views and in her private life. One of the few nursing leaders to marry and have a family, Robb demonstrated that it was possible to have both a public career and a private married life. Unfortunately, Robb's career as a prominent nursing leader ended abruptly when she died following a streetcar accident on April 15, 1910. However, prior to her death, Robb wrote her thoughts about the advances made in nursing during the thirty-five years of the modern nursing movement. In many places trained nurses were still regarded as "neither fish, flesh, nor fowl," and Robb told a story about passing two boys playing ball on the street. One of the boys shouted to the other, "Look out, you will hit that woman," and the other one replied, "She's not a woman, she's a nurse."[19]

Nursing's quintessential social reformer, feminist, suffragist, activist, educator, writer, and public health nurse Lavinia Dock epitomized the woman's movement in nursing. She completed her nurse training at Bellevue Hospital in New York in 1886, and by 1887 held a supervisory position at the hospital. After working at Bellevue for a few years, Dock became assistant superintendent of nurses at the Johns Hopkins Hospital in Baltimore in 1890. While at Johns Hopkins, Dock worked with superintendent and nursing leader Isabel Hampton [Robb] and met yet another future leader in nursing, Adelaide Nutting (1858–1948). Dock vigorously assisted in the formation of both the Superintendents' Society and the Associated Alumnae. Between 1896 and 1901, Dock served as secretary of the Superintendents' Society and authored many articles that supported the formation of the Associated Alumnae. Dock's interest in associations spread to the international nursing community, and in 1899 she helped organize the International

Council of Nurses and served as its first secretary. Of all the nursing leaders involved in professional associations, Dock most vocally appreciated the work of other women's clubs and organizations.[20]

Adelaide Nutting (1858–1948) served two terms as president of the Superintendents' Society in 1896 and again in 1909. She also spent two additional terms as secretary of the society in 1903 and 1905. Nutting's contribution to the Superintendents' Society included not only her many terms in executive positions but her visionary ideas throughout the years she acted as chair of the educational committee. In 1889, at the age of thirty-one, Nutting entered the newly opened nurse training school at the Johns Hopkins University. Following graduation in 1891, she worked as head nurse and later as assistant superintendent at the Johns Hopkins Hospital. When Isabel Hampton (Robb), superintendent of the school, married in 1894, Nutting replaced Hampton as the school's superintendent. Nutting proceeded to establish the Johns Hopkins school as one of the important nurse training schools in the country. In 1899, under the auspices of the Superintendents' Society, an advanced post-graduate course for nurses had been started at Teachers College, Columbia University in New York. In 1907, Nutting left her position at the John Hopkins to develop an expanded post-graduate course for nurses in hospital economics under the Department of Household Administration at Teachers College. While at Teachers College, Nutting earned the title as America's first professor of nursing. Nutting's interest in nursing displayed itself in her noted historical collection of nursing books and documents. This love for history prompted her famous four-volume book, *A History of Nursing,* coauthored with her colleague, Lavinia Dock, between 1907 and 1912. Nutting's interest in women's organizations extended beyond nursing and she helped found the American Home Economics Association as well as its *Journal of Home Economics* in 1908. She was also a member of the Cosmopolitan Club in New York City and a founder of the Women's Faculty Club of Columbia University.[21]

Annie Damer (1858–1915) served for five years as president of the Associated Alumnae between 1901–02 and 1905–1909. She graduated from the nurse training school at Bellevue Hospital in 1885, two years after Isabel Hampton Robb and one year before Lavinia Dock. Her organizational responsibilities included planning the logistical arrangements at the International Congress of Nurses held in September 1901 in Buffalo, New York. Interested in public health, Damer helped to establish a social service department for tuberculosis patients at Bellevue Hospital. Damer's strong leadership abilities continued to be demonstrated by the many executive positions she held in a variety of organizations. Not only did she preside over the Associated Alumnae, but she also served in similar roles for the American Journal of Nursing Company, the New York State Nurses' Association, and the Bellevue Nurses' Alumnae (1906–1908). She also actively worked toward uniting the Associated Alumnae with the American Red Cross. Following an accident in 1910, Damer's active professional life ended, but she was recognized for her pioneering leadership when in July 1914, the Associated Alumnae, now called the American Nurses Association (ANA), unanimously voted Annie Damer an honorary member.[22]

Another founder of the Superintendents' Society and the Associated Alumnae, Sophia Palmer (1853–1920), vigorously argued for social reform and nursing registration during her editorship of the Associated Alumnae's official journal, *The American Journal of Nursing*. She retained the position as the journal's first editor, held until she died in 1920. At twenty-two years of age, Palmer began her nursing training at the Boston Training School of Nurses (later known as Massachusetts General Hospital School of Nursing) where Linda Richards was superintendent. In addition to her editorship of the *AJN,* Palmer held several leadership positions in nursing following graduation from the training school in 1878. She served as charge nurse at Massachusetts General Hospital, superintendent of nurses at St. Luke's hospital in New Bedford, Massachusetts, and founder and director of a nurse training school at Garfield Memorial Hospital in Washington, D.C. Palmer, keenly aware of the power organizations generated, successfully involved the Federation of Women's Clubs in the Associated Alumnae's political battle to earn state nursing registration laws.[23]

One of the founding members and first president of the National Association of Colored Graduate Nurses (NACGN), Martha Minerva Franklin (1870–1968), served two years in office. Racial prejudice and discriminatory practices toward African-American nurses in the nursing profession preceded Franklin's monumental efforts to establish a new national nursing association. Between 1906 and 1908, Franklin studied the racially biased practices found in American nursing such as the exclusion of black women from most nurse training schools and the restrictive membership requirements in some state nurse associations, which in turn precluded membership in the American Nurses' Association. Franklin concluded from her study that a national association had to be formed in order to address the special needs of African-American nurses. In 1908, the first meeting of the NACGN convened in New York City. Franklin received her nurse training at the Women's Hospital Training School for Nurses of Philadelphia between 1895 and 1897 and she worked as a private duty nurse for several years. When Franklin relocated to New York City in 1920, she continued to further her education and attended a six-month post-graduate course at Lincoln Hospital in New York City. Between 1928 and 1930, at the age of fifty-eight, Franklin enrolled in graduate nursing education at Teachers College, Columbia University.[24]

The president of the NACGN between 1916–1923, Adah Belle Samuels Thoms (1870–1943), first worked as a schoolteacher in Richmond, Virginia, prior to entering nurse training. Thoms completed the nurse training course at the Woman's Infirmary and School of Therapeutic Massage in New York City in 1900 and found herself the only black student in a class of thirty women. After completing her basic nursing education at the Woman's Infirmary, Thoms wanted to improve her nursing education and entered the newly opened nurse training school for black women at Lincoln Hospital and Home in New York City. She graduated from Lincoln Hospital in 1905 and worked there for eighteen years as supervisor of nurses. Although Thoms served as acting director for the school between 1906 and 1923, she never was promoted to full director because racial discrimination prohibited her advancement. As founder and president of the Lincoln Nurses' Alumnae Association organized in 1903, she helped organize the NACGN and served as its first treasurer. Thoms became internationally involved in nursing in her position as one of the three NACGN delegates invited to attend the International Council of Nurses in 1912 in Cologne, Germany. She led the NACGN crusade to participate in the Red Cross nursing effort during World War I and continually advocated for the NACGN's affiliation with the National League of Nursing Education, the American Nurses Association, and the National Organization for Public Health Nursing. Thom's book, *The Pathfinders,* published in 1929, provides the first rich history of the African-American nurse in America.[25]

One of the originators of public health nursing in America and founder of the Henry Street Nurses Settlement in New York City in 1893, Lillian Wald (1867–1940), organized and served as the first president of the National Organization for Public Health Nursing (NOPHN) in 1912. Wald graduated in 1891 from the two year nurse training school at New York Hospital in New York City. Following graduation, Wald enrolled at the Women's Medical College and while there volunteered her nursing services to the new immigrants on New York City's lower east side. Greatly moved by the experiences she had while working in the community, Wald left medical school in 1893 and moved to the lower east side with another 1891 graduate nurse from the New York Hospital, Mary Brewster (1864–1901). Wald and Brewster served as visiting nurses, caring for the sick and teaching health-promoting behaviors and disease prevention to families in the community. Wald found financial backing for her venture from the Loeb and Schiff families, philanthropists who purchased the settlement house on Henry Street and paid the visiting nurses their salaries of $60 a month. A skilled fund-raiser, Wald raised enough money to increase the number of trained nurses working in the settlement house from nine trained nurses in 1893 to twenty-seven in 1907, and to more than 250 in 1916. By 1913 the Henry Street Settlement had a budget of more than $600,000 a year and had expanded services to seven different locations throughout New York City, with public health nurses making more than 1,300 visits a day to patients. Wald wrote of her experiences on the lower east side of New York in her books, *The House on Henry Street,* published in 1915, and *Windows on Henry Street,* published in 1934. Throughout the first half of the twentieth century, Wald spearheaded public health reforms such as the drives for better housing, child protection laws, formation of city parks, clean milk legislation, establishment of well baby clinics, and placement of nurses in public schools. She supported woman suffrage, advocated equal rights for women, and actively participated in the peace movement during World War I.[26]

Another founder and leader of the National Organization of Public Health Nursing (NOPHN), Ella Phillips Crandall (1871–1938), graduated nurse training in 1897 from a two-year course given at the General Hospital School in Philadelphia, Pennsylvania. During the early days of her career she worked in supervisory positions in hospitals in her hometown of Dayton, Ohio. She became active in public health nursing in 1909 when she became supervisor at the Henry Street Nurses Settlement, and in 1910 worked with Adelaide Nutting at Teachers College to develop courses in public health nursing at the college. Greatly influenced by Lillian Wald and Adelaide Nutting, Crandall actively pursued the formation of the NOPHN in 1912. Wanting to preserve the high standards of nursing practice in public health, Crandall, along with other public health nurses, helped to form the NOPHN. Crandall became the first executive secretary of the NOPHN following its creation on June 7, 1912. Noted for her administrative talents, Crandall established the NOPHN's national headquarters in New York City, hired a staff of more than twenty, and converted the quarterly magazine of the Cleveland Visiting Nurse Association into the official journal of the NOPHN, *Public Health Nurse*.[27]

Another pioneer in public health nursing, Mary Sewall Gardner (1871–1961), authored the well-known textbook, *Public Health Nursing*, in 1916 and served as the NOPHN's secretary in 1912 and as its president between 1913–1916. Gardner entered nurse training at the Newport Hospital Training School of Nurses in Newport, Rhode Island, in 1901 at the age of thirty. Following graduation in 1905, she held many leadership positions in nursing. Gardner worked in public health and actively sought continued improvement in the delivery of public health nursing. Her nursing interests extended to the international nursing community and she chaired the International Council of Nurses from 1925–1933.[28]

These names represent only a handful of the pioneer nursing leaders who spearheaded the drive for professional organization of nursing. Nurses created organizations specifically related to their special interests and needs. Superintendents who directed the graduate and student nurses at hospitals also served as the directors of the nurse training schools connected with the hospitals. In this dual role, superintendents focused on student nursing education while managing the nursing practice of hospital staff. Superintendents' responsibilities included teaching students as well as setting standards of admission, education, and graduation from the school. "Trained nurses," later called "graduate nurses," had completed a nurse training program and worked in hospitals either as a superintendent, supervisor, or assistant supervisor. Supervisors and assistant supervisors managed and instructed the nursing students; head nurses were responsible for the running of the hospital wards. However, this position was usually filled by a nursing student in her second or third year of training. Students in the first few months of training were called probationers. This period allowed students time to decide if nursing was the right career for them and it gave the school a chance to decide if the student was right for the work. Those graduate nurses who did not work in hospitals often worked as private duty nurses. The private duty nurse earned her salary by working in a patient's home and being paid by the family. Often, private duty nurses found their jobs through a nurses' directory run by a nurses' alumnae association, a hospital, a physician, or sometimes a pharmacy. However, as Louise Darche pointed out, good schools usually had a school registry which proved "a natural and legitimate connecting link between herself and the public."[29] A private duty nurse could expect to make from "$400 to $500 or even $600 yearly, over and above their board, washing, and lodging, and allow themselves a vacation of a couple of months every year."[30]

In 1912, Nutting described three general areas where trained nurses worked: in hospitals, as private duty nurses, and as visiting nurses in schools, factories, and the homes of the sick poor.[31] Visiting nurses, previously known as "district nurses" and later known as "public health nurses," worked outside of the hospital in the community. Initially, visiting nurses worked with families of the sick poor and then expanded their work to include families of the middle class. Public health nurses defined their nursing role to include teaching and promoting of preventative health care measures. They concerned themselves with public health problems such as reducing infant mortality, controlling communicable diseases in the community, and promoting healthy behaviors in families. Visiting nurses found themselves providing nursing care in the community well baby clinics, schools, and factories.[32]

Superintendents with responsibility for the education and training of nursing students who wanted to improve and control nursing education formed the Superintendents' Society in 1893. From their first meeting at the Chicago World's Fair, members of the Superintendents' Society talked about the formation of a national organization for all graduate nurses working in hospitals, private duty, or public health. Thus, the lack of state registration for nurses and the needs of working nurses gave impetus to the formation of the Nurses' Associated Alumnae in 1896. The National Association of Colored Graduate Nurses formed in 1908 to provide support and an organizational structure to

African-American nurses who in most instances experienced exclusionary practices in American nursing. The National Organization for Public Health Nursing convened for the first time in 1912 because visiting nurses wanted to control their own standards of practice in this emerging clinical setting. Thus, each nursing organization formed as a result of a predetermined need that only the strength of a group could overcome.[33]

These four nursing organizations shared common interests in nursing education, standards of practice, registration of nurses, and political and social reforms. The mostly female membership in nursing's four associations paralleled other late nineteenth and early twentieth-century women's reform groups such as the suffrage organizations, women clubs, and temperance leagues. However, nursing organizations directed their interests towards their professional growth and survival and thus related all social and political causes to their professional goals. For the Superintendents' Society, the Nurses' Associated Alumnae, the National Organization of Colored Graduate Nurses, and the National Organization for Public Health Nursing, nursing as a profession was a cause unto itself from which American society would ultimately benefit.

During the late nineteenth and early twentieth century, as nursing organizations arose in America, reform movements swept the country. To improve society and create a better world, people joined such Progressive Era movements as the settlement house movement, the suffrage movement, and the modern nursing movement. Women who joined these movements hoped to better their own lives and the lives of others by politically seeking personal and professional reform.[34] The modern nursing movement afforded women a professional opportunity to participate in social change and those who selected nursing as a career found that the nineteenth century women's issues were embedded in the twentieth century professional development of nursing. For many women who entered the profession, nursing provided a "window of opportunity."[35]

THE SUPERINTENDENTS' SOCIETY AND ITS IMPACT ON THE NURSING PROFESSION

America's progressive spirit of reform embraced by superintendents of the newly formed nurse training programs translated into organizational activities. Nursing superintendents created what is believed to be

America's first national professional women's organization, the American Society of Superintendents of Training Schools for Nurses, in 1893.[36] The concept of the Superintendents' Society, which in 1912 was renamed the National League of Nursing Education (NLNE), originated at the Nurses Congress, a subsection of the Hospital and Medical Congress held at the World's Columbian Exposition in Chicago in 1893.[37]

During the exposition, women for the first time played a significant role in original displays of sculpture, paintings, and "fancy work and in all the occupations."[38] The exposition's grounds and building committee decided that a woman should design the Woman's Pavilion and invited women to submit their plans in a contest. Twelve women submitted architectural drawings and the design of Bostonian Sophia G. Hayes won. The committee engaged Hayes to design and oversee the construction of the Woman's Pavilion. Bertha Honore Palmer (1849–1918), one of Chicago's most prominent socialites and social reformers, chaired the exposition's board of lady managers. She commended the board of directors for giving the board of lady managers full control of the Woman's Building and "all of the interests of women in connection with the Exposition." During the dedication ceremonies, Palmer highlighted a woman's grand opportunity to demonstrate her full breadth of intelligence and talent as "a more congenial companion and fit partner for her illustrious mate."[39]

As construction of the Woman's Pavilion in Chicago was underway, Ethel Bedford Fenwick (1857–1947), the well-known English nursing leader, was preparing her country's trained nurses' exhibit at the Woman's Pavilion.[40] Her interest in professionally organizing British nurses extended to trained nurses in America. In 1892, when Fenwick visited Chicago to work on the British exhibit during the winter before the fair opened, she suggested to the fair organizers that a nursing subsection be included among the International Congresses scheduled to convene at the fair. Following Fenwick's suggestion, chairman of the Hospital and Medical Congress of the International Congress of Charities, Correction and Philanthropy, Dr. Billings of Washington, formed a nursing subsection and invited the superintendent of the Johns Hopkins Hospital in Baltimore, Isabel Hampton, to chair the Nurses' Congress.[41]

The Nurses' Congress met for three days in June of 1893 in the Hall of Columbus in Chicago. Superintendents of training schools had traveled from throughout the United States and Canada to attend this notable meeting.[42] In an anthology of the papers and discussions from the International Congress of Charities, Correction, and Philanthropy, Isabel Stewart proclaimed that the 1893 World's Fair Congress on Hospitals, Dispensaries, and Nursing marked "the 'coming out' of nursing as a profession . . . ."[43] Each speech encouraged trained nurses to take charge of the emerging profession by organizing nursing associations at the local, state, national and international levels.

The chaotic conditions described in Isabel Hampton's opening address resulted from too many schools and too little professional control. Hampton demanded better educational standards in nursing and proposed ways to involve organized nursing in obtaining these standards. This seminal conference attracted the support of nursing's English heroine, Florence Nightingale, who prepared and sent her paper, "Sick Nursing and Health Nursing," to be read at the conference. American nursing leaders such as Lavinia Dock, Louise Darche, Irene Sutliffe (1850–1936), and Edith Draper (d. 1941) presented papers reflecting their vision of nursing to the congress as well. Draper's paper spoke directly, as her title suggested, to the "Necessity of an American Nurses Association," and she urged the formation of a national organization of graduated, trained nurses.[44]

During the Nurses' Congress, Hampton mobilized her colleagues to form a national association. Ever mindful of the woman movement's influence on nursing's development, Louise Darche, superintendent of the New York City Training School, said in her presentation, entitled, "Proper Organization of Training Schools in America," delivered during one of the sessions of the Nurses' Congress, that responsibility for the advancement of nursing belonged to women.[45]

Later that day, eighteen superintendents who had attended the Nurses' Congress met with the superintendent from New York City's St. Lukes Hospital, Katherine Lett (d. 1893), in her sitting room and formed a temporary association. Those in attendance elected the superintendent from Mount Sinai Hospital in New York, Anna Alston, as the temporary chair of the newly-formed association.[46] They also formed a committee that prepared the resolutions and bylaws that would govern and provide structure for the proposed society. The membership of the resolution committee consisted of six nursing leaders: Isabel Hampton; Mary P. Davis (1840?–1924)[47] from University Hospital in Philadelphia; Louise Darche; Mary McKechne of City Hospital in Louisville,

Kentucky; Sophia Palmer (1853–1920); Irene Sutliffe, superintendent of the New York Hospital Training School for Nurses; and Katherine Lett. This prestigious group founded the American Society of Superintendents of Training Schools for Nurses and drafted the governing constitution and bylaws for the newly formed society. The purpose of the Superintendents' Society was to "promote fellowship of members . . . to establish and maintain a universal standard of training . . . and . . . to further the best interests of the profession."[48] On June 15, 1893, the charter members of the temporary society present at the Chicago exposition unanimously adopted the founding committee's constitution and bylaw resolutions. When the Superintendents' Society held its first meeting the following January in New York, the superintendents who attended also ratified the resolutions of the temporary organization.

Forty-four superintendents attended the Superintendents' Society's first meeting on January 10 and 11, 1894, at the Academy of Medicine in New York City. Many had learned of the proposed society through an advertisement placed by the founding committee in the October 1893 issue of the journal, *Trained Nurse*. The published announcement invited all interested superintendents of nurse training schools in the United States and Canada to send their names, addresses, and hospitals to Anna Alston, president of the temporary Superintendents' Society. The announcement reported that the society's purpose was to "advance and perfect the practice of nursing and to elevate the profession."[49] From the printed invitation in *Trained Nurse,* only thirteen superintendents wrote to Alston they would attend. Undaunted by the low response, Alston obtained a listing of some seventy-one superintendents throughout the United States and Canada and sent each one an invitation to the January meeting. Forty-two responded to her invitation; twelve declined but stated they supported the proposed society, and thirty said they would attend.[50]

The first order of business on the agenda of the January 1894 meeting was the ratification of the constitution and bylaws that had been drafted at the 1893 Chicago exposition meeting. The constitution described four membership categories for the Superintendents' Society: active, associate, honorary, and corresponding. Active membership included all members of the preliminary association and "all past and present superintendents of training schools" from incorporated and well-organized general hospitals.[51] Each member had to be a "graduate in good and regular standing" from a nurse training school connected with a general hospital with no less than a two-year course.[52] Associate members included assistant superintendents who after two years could apply to the society's governing council for change to active membership status. The category of corresponding member was reserved for actively working trained nurses who did not live in the United States or British America, and honorary membership was reserved for boards of managers of training schools for nurses, trustees of hospitals, and others who showed an interest in advancing the nursing profession. According to the accepted bylaws, the association would hold annual meetings and charge an initiation fee of $5 from active members and $3 from associate members. In addition, every active and associate member would pay an "annual tax" not to exceed $3 for active members or $1 for associate members.[53]

During the afternoon session of January 10th, the superintendents heard three papers presented by two of their colleagues. Mary Littlefield, superintendent at the training school at Episcopal Hospital in Philadelphia, read the first two papers, "What is A Trained Nurse?" and "What are Nursing Ideals?" Lavinia Dock presented the third paper, "Non-Payment System as Established in the Illinois Training School." A discussion followed the reading of the papers and the issue of extending nurse training courses into a three-year program was raised. Most superintendents favored lengthening nursing programs in the abstract but believed that implementing this at their hospital schools was "practically almost impossible." As an outcome of the "lively" discussion that followed, the membership of the Superintendents' Society appointed Isabel Hampton, Lavinia Dock, and Lucy Walker, superintendent from Presbyterian Hospital Training School in Philadelphia, to a committee to study this proposal in conjunction with another proposal that would shorten students' work to an eight-hour day.[54]

On January 11, 1894, the second day of the meeting, members of the new association elected Linda Richards, superintendent at New England Hospital Training School in Boston, as president; Irene Sutliffe, superintendent of the New York Hospital Training School, as vice-president; Louise Darche as secretary; Lucy Drown (1848–1934), superintendent of the nurse training school at Boston City Hospital, as treasurer; Diane Kimber (?–1928), assistant superintendent of the New York City Training School on Blackwell's Island, and Ida Sutliffe, superintendent at the nurse training school at the Long Island College Hospital in Brooklyn, New York, as auditors; and as councilors, Isabel Hampton, G. Livingston, superintendent at Montreal General Hospital Training School, Montreal, Canada, Anna Maxwell (1851–1929), from Presbyterian Hospital, New York, Lavinia Dock, and Agnes Snively from Toronto General Hospital in Toronto, Canada.[55]

One of the agenda items on the second day was discussion about establishing a second national nursing association to be organized specifically for trained nurses from nurse training school alumnae associations throughout the United States and Canada. Isabel McIsaac (1858–1914), assistant superintendent of the Illinois Training School in Chicago, described to the superintendents at the meeting how nursing graduates had recognized the professional and personal benefits of organizing, and some had formed local alumnae associations at their training schools. Through these alumnae associations trained nurses found companionship and collegiality which had been lost to them after graduation.[56]

By 1894, more than six training school alumnae associations had been formed and many new ones originated over the next few years. Alumnae associations were a means of developing the ethics of nursing and formed the nuclei of club life for trained nurses. Moreover, local alumnae associations were to be the basis for a national alumnae association which the Superintendents' Society hoped to establish. The Superintendents' Society urged all training schools to establish alumnae associations, which in turn would join the national group that would become a national nurses alumnae association.[57]

The second annual conference of the Superintendents' Society in Boston on February 13th and 14th, 1895, continued to shape the goals of the association. In her address to the convention, Linda Richards, newly elected president, reflected on changes in nursing since her own first experience as a young administrator twenty years earlier. She described a "revolution of feeling toward training schools and trained nurses."[58] Although twenty years earlier the formally trained nurse had been considered undesirable by doctors, untrained nurses, and hospital board members, this new professional was now held in high regard. Richards remarked that to visit Bellevue, Blackwell's Island, and other hospitals revealed the positive effects of nurse training: "The perfect cleanliness and order of the yards, the homelike appearance, the contented faces of the patients, make even hospital workers wonder how so much can have been done."[59] In conclusion, Richards urged the Super-intendents' Society to continue their work to better the training of nurses in America.

Discussion about the organization of alumnae associations into a national group continued at the 1895 annual convention. The former superintendent of Garfield Memorial Hospital in Washington, D.C., Sophia Palmer (1853–1920), presented results of a survey she had taken in 1894 which looked at training schools and the formation of alumnae associations. Palmer's study focused on 164 training schools: 20 in Canada and 144 in the United States. Of the 109 schools that re-sponded, twenty-one schools had functioning alumnae associations or clubs with a printed constitution, ten had such groups in the process of organization, and seventy-eight had no organization but showed inter-est in establishing one. She classified the existing alumnae associations into three groups: (1) those organized and managed by alumnae of the training school; (2) those called nurses' clubs open to alumnae and stu-dents of other schools; and (3) religious societies open to alumnae and clergymen, officers, or members of the training school board.[60]

Palmer urged the superintendents at the convention to form alum-nae associations at their own schools for the purpose of gaining control and power. Members of the Superintendents' Society supported alum-nae associations as the means to organize individual trained nurses and harness their collective energy. Palmer argued that "organization is the power of the age. Without it nothing great is accomplished."[61] She urged this grass roots approach and encouraged even the smallest hospi-tal schools to start an association to ensure that trained nurses at all lev-els become involved in the social and political activities of the day and of their profession:

> *Remember that it is only through organization that individual mem-bers can be reached, and their co-operation in progressive movements be obtained, and that without their support and their good influence with the public we lose an immense power.*[62]

In one Superintendents' Society session, superintendent of the Toronto General Hospital Mary Agnes Snively (1848–1933), catego-rized the arguments of opponents to nursing education. In "A Uniform Curriculum for Training Schools," she stated that opposition to this nurse reform was based on the principle that a little knowledge was a dangerous thing and cautioned that those critics wanted nurses to re-main ignorant of current scientific knowledge and thus to continue to practice in the "mechanical fashion of a few years ago."[63] However, Snively asked her colleagues, "who will estimate the value of a nurse in charge of a class of enteric fever . . . who understands ulcerated condi-tion of the intestines and the importance of thorough cleanliness, venti-lation, and disinfection of excreta. . . ?"[64] Snively demanded a uniform curriculum that would be evaluated by uniform examinations and thus would assure higher quality among training school graduates, uphold a professional nursing standard and prevent the unqualified from calling themselves nurses. Not unlike the other professional groups of medicine and law, uniformity of professional accreditation for nursing was desir-able and obtainable. Moreover, Snively felt that professional graduation standards earned public respect for the nursing profession.[65]

During the fourth and final session of the Superintendents' Soci-ety's second annual convention, Lavinia Dock addressed the issue of control of private duty nursing in "Directories for Nurses." Directories assigned private duty nurses to their private duty cases and in most in-stances set the fees to be paid to the nurse by the family. However, Dock argued, "it should be for nurses themselves to fix the rates of pay-ment charged in private duty, and to state these rates to the registry—not the registry to the nurses."[66] She condemned the frequent practice of registries controlled by authorities other than nurses, whether they be neighborhood drugstores or the local medical society. Dock envi-sioned private duty nurses establishing and running their own directo-ries through professional nursing organizations. These nurse-run registries would self-regulate the fees for private duty nurses and would set standards of practice for them as well. Dock said that fees for the private duty nurse would be sensitive to the economic supply and de-mand for professional services and asked her colleagues to fully grant that nurses had a "perfect right to charge a higher rate than usual—if her opportunities or ability can command it."[67] Private duty nurses had to assert ownership of their economic livelihood by determining assign-ments and fees for private duty cases.

In the same speech, Dock advocated that women in nursing receive equal pay with men who nurse. It was common knowledge among the nurses that men who nursed, whether trained or untrained, com-manded higher rates than women. Men who were trained in nursing reportedly earned from $5 to $7 a day compared with women, who earned about \$3 a day.[68] Dock challenged the argument that women who worked for pay took jobs away from men who presumably financially supported dependents. Dock asserted that nursing was peculiarly women's work, thus no jobs were lost by men, and that most young men in nursing were not supporting families while many women in the profession had some financial responsibility for their families.[69]

Educational changes such as a standardized curriculum, a three-year training program, and a shorter eight-hour work day for pupil nurses remained major issues for the Superintendents' Society. Isabel Hampton [Robb] opposed the long ten- and twelve-hour work days required of pupil nurses in training. Their extended shifts served the needs of the hospital instead of the pupil's educational needs. She argued in favor of an eight-hour day to preserve the health of the students and to allow students time to pursue their studies. To support the argument to protect overburdened pupil nurses, Robb pointed to how leaders of the labor movement were advocating an eight-hour work day as reasonable for men. Robb asked how the public could demand more of women in nursing, who spent most of the time on their feet, their patience and temper enormously taxed, and who were "burdened with no little mental anxiety and responsibility."[70] Moreover, according to Robb, along with establishing a shorter work day for their pupil nurses, training schools needed to move to a three-year curriculum to replace the one- or two-year programs. Both reforms were necessary to preserve student health and ensure better education and training for graduate nurses.

Papers presented at the 1898 fifth annual convention of the Superintendents' Society reflected the membership's support for assisting superintendents to acquire the needed expertise to control the curriculum and administration of their nurse training schools. At the convention, Linda Richards clarified the duties of a superintendent as including instruction of pupil nurses, the care of patients in the hospital wards, management of the nurses' residence, and the discipline of pupil nurses. Often, superintendents were only responsible for the nurse training school, but in some institutions they had the dual job of administering the school and the hospital.[71] Superintendents found their job of educating pupil nurses fraught with opposition from hospital administrators, many of whom were businessmen or physicians who knew nothing of nursing or the proper education of nurses. While superintendents of some schools were in complete charge of nursing education, in other schools the education of nursing students remained in the hands of administrators who were uneducated in the art of nursing. Richards pointedly asked how an ordinary businessman or woman could "be a competent judge in training school matters?"[72] An unacceptable situation in any other practice, she challenged this intrusion into nursing which allowed well-trained professional women to be dominated by administrators who lacked nursing credentials.

Because the work of superintendents required skills that far exceeded the content of nurse training programs, Isabel Hampton Robb suggested that post-graduate training for such positions be established. According to Robb, in addition to an excellent understanding of nursing practice, a superintendent's role required a woman to have executive ability, an extensive liberal education, tact, refinement, and keen perceptions. Even if a trained nurse had all of the necessary characteristics required of the job of superintendent or nursing instructor, the newcomer had no exposure to the pedagogy of teaching nursing effectively. Thus, Robb believed that a training school for teachers, such as the one at Teachers College, Columbia University, in New York City was an appropriate place to initiate a post-graduate program for nursing. To fulfill one of the Superintendents' Society's chief objectives to "leave the work of nursing in a better condition than we found it," Robb proposed that the society establish a central board of Examiners who would set the requirements for post-graduate programs as well as assist in the development of new programs that prepared teachers and administrators of nursing.[73]

Following Robb's presentation, the Superintendents' Society passed a motion to appoint an education committee that would look into the establishment of a post-graduate course to educate trained nurses to teach nursing. The committee members included nursing superintendents and educators such as Linda Richards, Isabel Hampton Robb, Adelaide Nutting, Agnes Snively, and Lucy Drown.

Within a year, the committee's efforts yielded success: a course in hospital economics (as it was first called) opened to two students in 1899 at Teachers College, Columbia University. One of the two students, Anna Alline (1864–1934), later worked in the school's post-graduate nursing program. Those enrolled in nursing's first one-year course in home economics took courses in psychology, education, biology, physical science, and social science, including one course entitled "Social Reform Movements." The superintendents on the education committee strongly advocated the study of social reforms, recognizing that "our schools touch these problems constantly and the superintendents need to know more about them that they may take advantage of that knowledge . . . ."[74] Mary Adelaide Nutting, one of the committee members, noted that all professors, teachers, and thoughtful people found the "problem of social reform a burning one."[75] The Superintendents' Society supported the program with financial contributions, by giving educational expertise, and by volunteering faculty such as Lavinia Dock and Lillian Wald, who had developed specialized nursing expertise in social reform and public health.[76]

Mary Adelaide Nutting became the head of the new Department of Household Administration at Teachers College at Columbia University in 1907 where she earned a reputation as a leading educator in nursing education in America and was the first graduate nurse to hold the title of professor of nursing. At that time, the philanthropist and friend to nursing, Helen Hartley Jenkins (1860–1934), donated $200,000 to endow a new department of nursing and health at Teachers College. During the formative years after the turn of the century, the Superintendents' Society referred often to the nursing program at Teachers College as a source of pride and achievement in its efforts to nurture the development of new educators in nursing. Thus, knowledge through formal education, as well as on-the-job experience that fostered expertise, became the powerful tools used by nursing superintendents and instructors to claim and gain control of curriculum in the years to come.[77]

To raise the standards of nursing education and practice, the Superintendents' Society continued work toward establishing a national association of alumnae organizations. To this end it began the Nurses' Associated Alumnae of the United States and Canada (hereafter called the Associated Alumnae) in 1896.

THE NURSES' ASSOCIATED ALUMNAE OF THE UNITED STATES AND CANADA AND THE CONCERNS OF WOMEN IN THE NURSING PROFESSION

As the number of hospital schools of nursing increased, the number of trained nurses rose steadily from 157 graduates in 1880, to 471 in 1890, and more significantly to 3,456 in 1900.[78] This group of working women had a unique set of needs related to job satisfaction, financial security, professional credentialing, and academic accreditation of schools. Trained nurses advocated state registration of graduate nurses to ensure that only trained professionals could use the title of "nurse." Cognizant of the increasing number of trained nurses and their special needs in practice, visionary nursing leaders had anticipated the formation of the Associated Alumnae three years earlier at the Chicago exposition in 1893.[79]

Later known as the American Nurses' Association (ANA), the Associated Alumnae formed in response to the needs of the growing number of trained nurses who were graduates from nurse training schools. While the Superintendents' Society limited its active membership to superintendents, the Associated Alumnae planned to recruit graduates of training schools into its membership.[80]

At the Superintendents' Society's second convention in 1895, a steering committee of twelve superintendents formed for the purpose of merging individual school alumnae associations into one national organization. Assisted by Lavinia Dock, the twelve-woman committee organized the alumnae association. Dock assumed the task of studying the issue of forming this second national association and presented her findings at the Superintendents' Society's 1896 third annual convention in a paper titled "A National Association for Nurses and Its Legal Organization." Dock examined the structure, governance, and goals of the national governments of the United States and Canada to discern how they influenced the development of national philanthropic and professional associations and labor unions.[81]

Dock studied organizational patterns of late nineteenth- and early twentieth-century reform groups such as the Woman's Christian Temperance Union, the International Brotherhood of Locomotive Engineers, Association of Collegiate Alumnae, and the American Medical Association to guide the Superintendents' Society plan for the new national nurses' alumnae association. Like these other reform groups, she envisioned a three-tier pattern of organization for nursing: the national nursing association responsible for developing the moral, ethical, and overriding principles for graduate nurses; state nursing associations concerned with the credentialing of graduate nurses and other state legislative issues which affected their work; and the local alumnae associations fostering collegiality among nursing alumnae, administering nursing registries, and supporting graduate nurses.[82]

Dock observed that it would take time to establish this working national nursing organization because individual nurse training schools first had to establish a network of local alumnae associations. The emergence of state nursing organizations required at least a five-year period in which to incorporate the local alumnae associations into a state-wide group, and finally one state would have to be selected in order for a national charter to be granted to a national organization.[83] Dock cautioned the Superintendents' Society that:

> *the growth of such a common feeling of loyalty to our work and responsibility toward one another as we need to cultivate is a slow one, not to be hastened, but to be fostered through years with painstaking care; that radical changes are not to be brought about in a day, and that reforms that are worth anything have to be worked for long and arduously.*[84]

Dock considered the argument for including training school board members who lacked nursing credentials as voting members in a national nursing organization, but after much consideration she supported including only trained graduate nurses into such an organization. She favored ex-officio status for non-nurse members which enabled them to debate, but not to vote. In this way, Dock felt that the ". . . benefits of a mixed membership might be reached, and the drawbacks avoided."[85]

In the same address Dock stressed the importance of differentiating a national nursing association from trade unions. She preferred that the proposed future national nursing association adhere to principles similar to those of other professional and educational reform groups rather than ally with the financial interests espoused by trade unions.

The superintendents approved of Dock's ideas and agreed that alumnae associations should be organized into a national organization which would include nurses from different training schools throughout the United States and Canada. Five members of the Superintendents' Society were appointed to organize a constitutional convention and write the constitution and bylaws for the proposed Nurses' Associated Alumnae which was to serve independent professional women who hoped by organization "to work many reforms."[86] The steering committee included Lavinia Dock as chairman and secretary of the constitutional convention; Isabel McIsaac; Isabel Merritt, superintendent from Brooklyn City Training School in Brooklyn, New York; M.B.

Brown, superintendent of Massachusetts General Training School, and Lucy Walker. The Superintendents' Society instructed them to select an additional fourteen delegates to their committee: one group of seven trained nurses and an additional seven who were members of the oldest alumnae societies and who did not hold hospital positions. This group formed the core of the constitutional convention designated to frame a national constitution for the alumnae association.

The constitutional convention was held September 2 and 4, 1896, at the Manhattan Beach Hotel in Brooklyn, New York.[87] The minutes of the Constitutional Convention which convened in Brooklyn indicate that twelve delegates from alumnae associations of training schools for nurses met with twelve members of the Superintendents' Society to plan the new organization. Delegates who attended the Brooklyn conference represented training school alumnae associations from the following hospital-based schools: Massachusetts General in Massachusetts; Presbyterian in New York; Bellevue in New York; Yale-New Haven in Connecticut; Orange Memorial in New Jersey; Johns Hopkins in Maryland; the University of Pennsylvania and Philadelphia in Pennsylvania; Brooklyn City Hospital in Brooklyn, New York; Illinois Hospital in Illinois, and the Farrand at Harper Hospital in Detroit, Michigan.[88]

At the Brooklyn meeting, the steering committee agreed to name the new organization the Nurses' Associated Alumnae of the United States and Canada, and proceeded to write its constitution and bylaws.[89] Steering committee members proposed that the new association should establish and maintain a code of ethics for nursing, elevate the standard of nursing education, promote the usefulness, honor, and interests of the nursing profession, inform the public to the work of nursing, and foster loyalty and friendly exchange among nurses. Membership eligibility served as de facto accreditation of the member's training school alumnae association: a local association must represent schools with no less than two full years of training and be affiliated with a hospital that maintained no less than fifty beds. The alumnae association required local chapters to pay an initiation fee of $5 for every twenty-five members; chapters with less than twenty-five members paid only $5. Moreover, the steering committee required no less than three alumnae associations within a state to allow organization of a state society.[90]

The steering committee set a date for the next meeting of the Nurses' Associated Alumnae for the "second Thursday and Friday in

February, 1897," at the same time the Superintendents' Society was to meet in Baltimore, Maryland, for their fourth annual meeting.[91] A newspaper clipping published one week before the Superintendents' Society's fourth annual meeting announced the formation of the Nurses' Associated Alumnae and stated its purpose to be "both ethical and educational."[92] At that meeting delegates from different alumnae associations and members of the steering committee voted to ratify the new constitution and bylaws of the Associated Alumnae.

The first annual convention of the Nurses' Associated Alumnae was held April 28–29, 1898, in New York City. In 1898, 23 nurse alumnae associations constituted the Associated Alumnae members; by 1912, that number increased to 142 alumnae associations and included 31 states, 24 county associations which together represented between 17,000 and 20,000 individual members. Members voted to change the name of the association to the American Nurses' Association in 1911.

At that first meeting in New York City, members discussed crucial issues regarding the policy and procedures of the new organization. They engaged in one of the first political struggles the organization faced when they discussed the Associated Alumnae's responsibility to supply trained nurse services to the government during the Spanish-American War (1898).[93] The United States had declared war on Spain one week prior to the Associated Alumnae's first meeting in New York. The army had not maintained a trained nursing service. The men who worked in the existing Army Hospital Corps provided the army with its "nurses," but they had little or no nurse training. Following the Civil War, women were not permitted to serve as trained nurses in the hospital corps and the surgeon-general of the army, George M. Sternberg, at the beginning of the Spanish-American War, wanted to uphold that precedent. However, realizing the increased demand that war would place on nurse services, Sternberg first allowed women to be nurses and dieticians only at base hospitals. When the need for nursing reached critical levels later that year, he yielded and finally authorized female nurses to be sent directly to the camps to care for the wounded and the sick.[94]

When America declared war on Spain, many women, including nurses, both trained and untrained, offered their services to the army. At the outset of the Spanish-American War, Anita Newcomb McGee (1864–1940), a physician and Washington socialite, offered her services and those of the Daughters of the American Revolution to screen nursing applicants for the army. General Sternberg appointed McGee as acting assistant surgeon-general to decide on nurse qualifications and placement of nurses in military service. A few days after the declaration of war, the Associated Alumnae, following their first annual meeting in New York in April 1898, contacted the secretary of war in Washington requesting permission to discuss the Associated Alumnae's plan to offer essential nursing services to the war effort. However, McGee and the Daughters of the American Revolution had already been assigned the job of accepting nurse applications and placement of nurses in the war.[95]

The issue of the Associated Alumnae's participation in America's war effort raised at the first annual meeting in April 1898, continued at a board meeting held on December 28, 1898. Under the direction of the association's president, Isabel Hampton Robb, the board met with the New York Training School to propose legislation which would lead to the professional control of a permanent Army Nurse Corps. The rationale for this was that the Associated Alumnae represented the largest organization of trained nurses and thus should monitor the work and control the entrance of trained nurses in the army.[96]

Initially McGee screened all applicants and accepted only trained nurses. However, due to the tremendous need for nurses, she set aside that policy and accepted untrained nurses and nurses who trained at schools that did not meet the professional standards of the Superintendents' Society or the Associated Alumnae. Robb, with the support of the Associated Alumnae, wanted to correct the misuse of untrained nurses and the poor supervision of trained ones. In hopes of rectifying the situation, the Associated Alumnae worked in collaboration with a group of independent Red Cross workers in New York who had formed the American Red Cross Relief Committee.[97] Both the Associated Alumnae and the American Red Cross Relief Committee worked toward establishing an Army Nurse Corps for trained nurses. However, political conflict within the American Red Cross, the already established control of army nursing by McGee and the Daughters of the American Revolution, and the newness of the Nurses' Associated Alumnae kept full control of army nursing during the Spanish-American War outside of the professional nursing organization.[98]

Although the professional organization did not officially participate in the war, they did supply some of the trained nurses that served. Individual members of the Associated Alumnae sent their applications to the surgeon-general and were selected to serve as nurses during the war.

In July 1898, Anna Maxwell (1851–1929), charter member of the Superintendents' Society, the Associated Alumnae, and the International Council of Nurses while superintendent of Presbyterian Hospital in New York, took leave from her position and organized the trained nurses sent to Camp Thomas, Chickamauaga Park, Georgia. Like Nightingale during the Crimean War, Maxwell found conditions in Georgia unsanitary, overcrowded, and inadequate to serve the wounded and sick soldiers at the camp. More than 50,000 soldiers living in the camp were exposed to an outbreak of measles; many had contracted yellow fever, typhoid fever, and malaria and needed the trained nurses. Maxwell was given authority by the surgeon-general to recruit trained nurses to work in the camp and the American Red Cross assisted her in the recruitment efforts. Her efforts and the work of the trained nurses improved conditions at the camp, reducing the mortality rate to only 67 deaths among 1,000 hospitalized patients.[99]

At the Associated Alumnae's third annual convention held in New York City in May 1900, Isabel Hampton Robb addressed the problems the organization faced during the Spanish-American War. In her opening address, Robb spoke of how the events over the past two years clearly confirmed the need for trained nurses to organize so they could promote protective legislation for nurses and patients. She said nursing had paid a price for organizing too late to be effective during the Spanish-American war ". . . for one can hardly doubt the nursing of our soldiers during the Spanish-American war would have naturally fallen in our hands had our organization been completed earlier."[100] As a result of this, the nursing profession endured opposition from people outside the nursing profession who were "purely commercial"[101] and who did not share the nursing profession's "high aims or definite principles."[102] The opposition's leaders were not trained nurses and the "success of their projects would mean the complete subjection of trained nurses."[103] Thus, Robb concluded that between the opposition and the professional nursing organization, no common ground existed which could facilitate compromise. Until trained nurses could take care of their own affairs they should not:

> *permit themselves to be guided and governed by women whose ruling motive must be a commercial one, as such women cannot appreciate the work to be done or the proper methods for performing it, as can trained nurses themselves.[104]*

Robb's presidential address at the third annual convention referred to the Army Nurse Corps legislation that would keep the work of trained nurses in the hands of trained nurses. Not only would they as a national organization continue to support the passage of the Army Nurse Corps bill, which would place trained nurses under the control of trained nurses, but each state nursing organization must continue to support state nurse registration laws. In hopes of strengthening Associated Alumnae efforts to achieve professional credentialing and recognition, Robb urged American nurses to unite with nursing professionals from other countries and to "become identified with woman's work at large all over the world."[105]

THE ASSOCIATED ALUMNAE AND THE SUPERINTENDENTS' SOCIETY AFFILIATE AS THE AMERICAN FEDERATION OF NURSES

By 1901 America's two newly established professional nursing organizations, the Superintendents' Society and the Nurses' Associated Alumnae, along with other women's groups, affiliated with the International Council of Women (ICW), the National Council of Women (NCW), and the International Council of Nurses (ICN). The merger of America's two nursing organizations into the American Federation of Nurses (AFN), enabled American nurses to be duly represented in the national and international women's organizations that had already formed in 1888.

The ICW had met for the first time in March 1888 in Washington, D.C., to celebrate the 40th anniversary of the Woman's Rights Convention of 1848. Women from fifty-three national organizations and forty-nine delegates from England, France, Denmark, Norway, Finland, India, Canada, and the United States were represented at that first meeting. As a result of that meeting, two councils of women emerged: an International Council of Women and a National Council of Women. The membership of the ICW consisted of national councils from different countries which represented numerous women's organizations involved in social, intellectual, moral or civic progress and reform. The founders of the ICW included leaders in many of the late nineteenth-century women's reform organizations such as suffragists Susan B.

Anthony and Elizabeth Cady Stanton; temperance leader and suffragist Frances Willard (1839–1898); May Wright Sewall (1844–1920), educator and advocate for world peace, social hygiene, woman suffrage, dress reform, and women's clubs; and Clara Barton (1821–1912), leader of the American Red Cross.[106]

The National Council of Women also organized in 1888 in Washington, D.C., and formed a means to link American women throughout the world with the ICW. The NCW served as a clearing house for exchanging information on activities of other national women's organizations in America. The idea for the national council originated with suffragist Elizabeth Cady Stanton early in the 1880s. Stanton proposed that an international group of women who supported woman suffrage be organized. Stanton found support for her idea from other late nineteenth-century women activists. Susan B. Anthony and May Wright Sewall with Frances Willard, first president of the National Council of Women, expanded on Stanton's idea to include all activities of organized womanhood regardless of their support of woman suffrage. May Wright Sewall and the corresponding secretary of the National Woman Suffrage Association, Rachel Foster Avery, further developed the plan for the National and International Councils of Women that subsequently became a reality in March, 1888. The comprehensive membership of the women's groups enabled the ICW and the NCW to keep abreast of "women's movements throughout the world."[107]

Ten years later, the International Council of Nurses was formed by the Matron's Council of Great Britain and Ireland (hereafter called the Matron's Council) and met for the first time at the International Council of Women quinquennial meeting held in London in 1899. While the ICW convened in London, trained nurses from America, Canada, Australia, Denmark, and Holland who attended the international women's congress met at the invitation of English nursing organizer Ethel Gordon Fenwick. Fenwick, with the British nursing organization, the Matron's Council of Great Britain and Ireland, had taken the initial steps to form nursing's international council. The Matron's Council had been formed in 1894 by English superintendents who staunchly supported English nurses' drive for registration. Fenwick extended her invitation to all international nursing delegates that attended the ICW. Although the goals of the ICW and the ICN were similar, the International Council of Nurses permitted American nursing to concentrate on world wide nursing issues and still address the general issues all women faced.[108]

The Superintendents' Society, at its fourth annual convention held in Baltimore, Maryland, in 1897, had received and read Fenwick's invitation to participate in the formation of an International Council of Nurses and to prepare a nurses' exhibit for the International Council of Women to be held in London in 1899. At the Baltimore meeting, the Superintendents' Society decided to send two representatives to the proposed international congress of nurses. Edith Draper (d. 1941) and a Miss Smith, both of whom had plans to visit England that summer, were selected to confer with the Matron's Council to discuss the proposed international nursing organization. However, at the Superintendents' Society's fifth annual convention held the following year in 1898, president Agnes Snively from Toronto, Canada, said that the Superintendents' Society governing council had met and agreed with regret that it would be too expensive to send a delegate or an exhibit to represent American nursing at the international conference to be held in London that year. Nevertheless, the international group of nurses met at the Matron's House at St. Bartholomew's Hospital in London and proceeded to write the constitution for an International Council of Nurses in 1899. "Self-government"[109] characterized the spirit and goal of the ICN. Meeting nurses throughout the world not only allowed greater communication among them but also deepened "sympathy" and made them "greater human beings."[110]

The president of the Superintendents' Society, Isabel McIsaac, received a letter dated December 17, 1898, from May Wright Sewall explaining why the society should consider membership in the NCW and subsequently the ICW. In her letter, Sewall explained that the primary objective of the NCW was to ". . . promote the advancement of human society through the enlargement of the recognition of women in various industries and professions."[111] Thus, Sewall explained it seemed only natural that the Superintendents' Society "should be affiliated with other organizations in the Council."[112]

The superintendents discussed Sewall's invitation to join the NCW at the sixth annual convention but made no decision at that time. However, a motion to join was finally passed at the seventh annual meeting following a discussion of membership in the NCW and the formal establishment of the International Council of Nurses at the seventh annual convention of the Superintendents' Society held in 1900 in Buffalo, New York.[113]

During the seventh annual meeting, the superintendents discussed several reasons why they should join the NCW and referred to a suggestion made by Sewall mentioned in another letter addressed to a member of the provisional committee, Lavinia Dock, dated February 23, 1900. The superintendents carefully considered the Sewall suggestion to enter the NCW as a joint venture with the newly formed Associated Alumnae. They also weighed Sewall's explanation of the differences between the ICW and the proposed ICN. Sewall pointed out to the superintendents that membership within the ICW could be achieved only through membership in the NCW and membership through another international organization was prohibited. Although an international affiliation with other nurses would be helpful to American nurses, Sewall questioned if this would provide nurses with the direct participation in the ICW. Sewall hoped that the Superintendents' Society would affiliate with the ICW, and in this way, nurses from many nations would be better served.[114]

Although the superintendents passed the resolution to join the National Council of Women at their seventh annual meeting, they continued to debate the importance of membership in the proposed International Council of Nurses. The appendix of the published minutes that year included three items on this matter: the National Council of Women's invitation to join; extracts from a draft constitution of the International Council of Women; and an extract of a letter from Ethel Fenwick. In the invitation to join the National Council of Women, an analogy between the "Industrial Machine" and the National Council of Women was made. The national council existed to serve as "the engine" for its member organizations and to "unite and concentrate scattered forces and amalgamate them into one."[115] Extracts from the draft constitution of the International Council of Nurses clearly stated the council's intention to promote international communication between nurses; the extracts also included the International Council of Nurses' proposal to plan a "quinquennial Congress of Nurses" to be held at the same time and place of the quinquennial meeting of the International Council of Women.[116]

The ICN envisioned that trained nurses would benefit from meeting other women workers throughout the world. Although membership within the ICN would sufficiently afford American nurses with such opportunities, the memorandum printed in the appendix of the superintendents' seventh annual convention indicated the only way to join the International Council of Women was through the National Council of Women in each country.[117]

Fenwick supported the Superintendents' Society membership in the NCW in a speech she presented at the conference of the Matron's Council held in London, July 1, 1899, which was published in the appendix of the proceedings of the seventh annual convention. Fenwick explained that since the exclusion of other international societies was not the purpose of the ICW, membership in the newly proposed ICN required that the respective national professional nursing groups join their country's NCW first.[118]

The Superintendents' Society had agreed at the seventh annual convention to affiliate with the NCW and subsequently the ICW. The mechanism for its entrance into the National Council of Women required some planning with the larger and newer nursing organization in America, the Associated Alumnae. In 1899, just two years after the Associated Alumnae had formed and eleven years after the founding of the ICW, Fenwick invited members of the Associated Alumnae to attend the meetings of the ICW. The Associated Alumnae read a letter received from Fenwick at the second annual convention of the Associated Alumnae held at the Academy of Medicine in New York City on May 1st and 2nd, 1899. Fenwick's letter invited American nurses to attend the meetings of the ICW. The following year, the Associated Alumnae, at its third annual convention held during May 1900, officially voted to affiliate with other women's organizations through membership in the ICW.[119]

Isabel Hampton Robb spoke at the 1900 convention and urged nurses to unite with women's groups throughout the world.[120] A member of the provisional committee, Lavinia Dock, also spoke and explained how the ICW had held its first quinquennial at the Columbian Exposition in Chicago in 1893, the same year the Superintendents' Society was founded.[121] From Dock, the members of the Associated Alumnae learned that eligibility to join the ICW required membership in America's NCW. Dock proposed that an affiliation between the Associated Alumnae and the Superintendents' Society would enable the members of both national nursing organizations to join the NCW. President of the NCW (1897–1899) and later president of the ICW

(1899–1904), May Wright Sewall wrote a letter to the Associated Alumnae that Dock read at the third annual convention. Sewall, in her letter, suggested that American nurses would be politically stronger if they entered the NCW as one united organization. In addition, Sewall explained it would be "much cheaper" to do this because the triennial fee for the NCW was $100. If one umbrella professional nursing organization represented the two existing nursing organizations, the membership cost to the Superintendents' Society and the Associated Alumnae would be shared and thus reduced.

During the Associated Alumnae's third annual convention, Lavinia Dock introduced the history of the newly formed ICN. At that meeting, President Robb asked Dock if the Associated Alumnae could join the ICN without joining the NCW. Dock responded that it was "of logical necessity that they hang together."[122] Dock explained further that "we can only share in the quinquennial, where our International Council of Nurses will meet, by belonging to the National Council of our country."[123]

The members of the Associated Alumnae continued to discuss at their meeting in 1900 the proposed affiliation of their association with the Superintendents' Society so they could join the National Council of Women and subsequently the International Council of Nurses. Robb asked Dock if the Superintendents' Society had considered joining the Associated Alumnae in this matter. Dock replied that while no decision had been made, the Superintendents' Society had already discussed affiliating with the alumnae association. Following discussion on this issue, a motion passed to form a committee to consider and to later report on the subject of affiliation between the Associated Alumnae and the Superintendents' Society for the purpose of joining the National Council of Women.[124]

During the third session of the 1900 convention, the chair of the committee to study the possible union with the NCW, Jessie Breeze, read a resolution that called for the merger of the Associated Alumnae and the Superintendents' Society in order to apply for membership to the National Council of Women and to the International Council of Women. Breeze also motioned that an appointment of two members from both the Superintendents' Society and the Associated Alumnae as well as two members-at-large be made and that the chair of the committee report back to both organizations yearly. The Associated Alumnae carried the resolution proposed. Dock assured the Associated

Alumnae that the Superintendents' Society wanted to affiliate so it could participate in the ICW.[125]

The Superintendents' Society and the Associated Alumnae, in a marriage of convenience, formed an umbrella organization using the name American Federation of Nurses (AFN) in 1901. Adelaide Nutting was elected president to serve a term of five years. The federation represented the membership of America's professional nursing organizations at the NCW and subsequently at the International of Congress of Women until the federation withdrew from the NCW in 1905. In spite of its withdrawal from the NCW, the federation continued to represent American nurses at the ICN until 1912. By the time the AFN held its first annual meeting in May 1905, in Washington, D.C., during the Superintendents' Society's eighth annual convention, the federation already had sent delegates to three annual meetings of the National Council of Women in Buffalo, 1901; Washington, 1902; and Indianapolis, 1904. The federation had also represented American nursing at the ICW quinquennial held in Berlin in 1905.[126]

Trained nurses in their individual alumnae associations acknowledged the importance of membership in the National Council of Women. In 1901, the secretary of the Alumnae Association of the Training School of Nurses of the New York Post-Graduate Medical School and Hospital, Mary E. Thornton, sent a letter to the graduating class of 1901 which reflected the progressive spirit of its members. Thornton, an 1890 graduate of the school urged new graduates to join the school's alumnae association and be eligible to attend the ICN meeting that would be held in Buffalo, New York, on September 6, 1901. In addition, she explained to the class of 1901 that, "there, too, we shall have for the first time representation in the National Council of Women. . . . Surely you will want to take part in this history-making epoch of your profession."[127]

On September 16th and 17th, 1901, the eighth annual meeting of the Superintendents' Society was held at the Women's Industrial Union in Buffalo. Lavinia Dock reported that through the newly formed AFN, the society had paid its dues and had joined the NCW.[128] The Superintendents' Society convention coincided with the 1901 Pan-American Exposition in Buffalo which attracted several international congresses. Emma Keating, the Superintendents' Society president and delegate to the NCW meeting, attended the National Council of Women and reported on the activities at the September 16th meeting.

Keating included in her report debates on resolutions demanding the appointment of women to public commissions specifically related to marriage and divorce, the decrease in immigration, and tax exemptions for church properties. Keating's report concluded by saying that the work of the NCW was 'interesting and instructive" but too time-consuming for women in nursing who had so much to accomplish in their own profession. Nonetheless, nursing representation continued in the NCW until 1905 when the AFN decided to drop its membership in the national council and focus its attention on the ICN.[129]

The AFN represented American nurses to other women's organizations who also belonged to the National and International Council of Women; thus, the federation provided a vehicle in which nursing could communicate to other women the advances made in the profession since 1873. This allowed the federation to seek backing for needed nursing legislation from affiliated women's groups in the National and International Council of Women.

In February 1904, one year before the federation resigned from the NCW, Helena Barnard from St. Joseph, Missouri, a graduate of the Johns Hopkins Hospital School for Nurses, represented the AFN at a meeting of the Executive Council of Women at Indianapolis. Barnard explained the history of the Superintendents' Society and the Associated Alumnae. She stressed the importance of the new legislation already passed in thirteen states requiring completion of a systematic course in nurse training and passage of a state examination before a nurse could use the new title of "registered nurse." Barnard asked the women's council to support the American nursing federation's continued efforts in creating this legislation to safeguard the public from unscrupulous schools and untrained nurses. She urged them "in conformity with the ever-growing spirit of philanthropy," to join American nurses in their work to "meet the needs of the day."[130] Barnard asked the societies affiliated with the National Council of Women to "support everywhere the nurse in her effort to secure legislation."[131]

In spite of the inroads made by the AFN's membership in the NCW, nursing leaders believed that they could more effectively communicate their professional concerns with other women in the international community through the International Council of Nurses. In 1905, the *Washington Post* announced that the AFN had withdrawn from the NCW, but had adopted a resolution "providing that the federation affiliate with the International Council of Nurses."[132] Dock explained why the AFN dropped its membership in the National Council of Women: the National Council of Women was ineffective as a national organization; dues were six times higher than other national councils; membership responsibilities were an added burden for the already busy officers of the professional nursing organizations; and membership in the ICN brought greater benefits to American nurses. Dock concluded that although membership in the National Council of Women was theoretically desirable, the limited resources of nursing leaders required that nursing organizations focus their energies on their members' professional concerns. Although Dock believed that they could be "definitely helpful and useful in an international union of our colleagues,"[133] she personally felt that the membership in the NCW had enabled them to "come into relation with nurses of other countries," and gave them "status in the great Congresses of Women."[134] Nevertheless, affiliation with the International Council of Nurses would continue the ties American nursing had already established with the early twentieth-century woman's movement.[135]

The AFN enabled American nurses to engage in and support the drive of late nineteenth- and early twentieth-century woman's movement for woman suffrage. The support of woman suffrage evolved as nurses learned of the relevance suffrage had for the profession, for the health of their patients, and for their personal lives. The AFN represented nurses' views on the suffrage question at the international council until the Associated Alumnae reorganized in 1911 and became the American Nurses' Association. Following this change, the American Nurses' Association in 1912 represented American nursing in the international community of nurses and endorsed an international professional nursing woman suffrage resolution.[136]

ASSOCIATED ALUMNAE ESTABLISH THE *AMERICAN JOURNAL OF NURSING*

Recognizing the need to communicate with the international nursing community, the Nurses' Associated Alumnae had joined the AFN. The Associated Alumnae believed that contact with other nurses internationally would ultimately lead to unity and strength among nurses in their drive to legitimize the profession of nursing by passage of worldwide nurse registration laws. Similarly, the Associated Alumnae pursued opportunities to facilitate communication among trained nurses in America in hopes of influencing the future development of the nursing profession in this country. The members of the Associated Alumnae were trained nurses, some of whom worked as private duty nurses, and others who worked in supervisory and teaching positions at hospitals. These nurses joined the Associated Alumnae for personal and professional benefits, to share the burdens of their daily work, and to improve the conditions of that work. In their state associations, nurses worked to achieve nursing registration through state-by-state legislation. However, the Associated Alumnae needed a means through which to speak out on the issues and concerns of professional nurses as well as to facilitate communication regarding the rapid changes nursing and health care experienced during the early years of the twentieth century.

Aware of the need to reach an increasing number of trained nurses from different states, different schools, and practice settings, the Associated Alumnae, with the help of the Superintendents' Society, established the professional periodical *American Journal of Nursing,* in 1900.[137] Founded by members of both the Superintendents' Society and the Associated Alumnae, the journal became the "mouth-piece for those societies, a bond of union between scattered nurses, and a means of education."[138] Sophia Palmer, superintendent of the Rochester City Hospital and first editor of the proposed journal, and Mary E. P. Davis, superintendent of the University of Pennsylvania Hospital, contributed the initial organization required to establish the journal. The Associated Alumnae established a journal committee, whose first members included Isabel Hampton Robb, Adelaide Nutting, and a Miss Harrington. The committee expanded as Mary E. P. Davis, who became chair, replaced Miss Harrington, and a Miss Stevenson of Boston, Sophia Palmer, and Harriet Fulmer of Chicago were added.[139]

During that year, Mary E. P. Davis devoted much time, energy and money to the planned publication. Davis sent out more than 5,000 letters, which secured 550 paid subscriptions for the publication's premier issue in October 1900. Also, Davis donated her time and underwrote the cost of the mailings, and raised pledges of more than $2,300 from alumnae associations, each of which advanced $100 or more to the project.[140]

A unique feature of the new nursing journal related to the control and ownership of the periodical by nursing professionals. The journal committee and the newly appointed first editor of the *AJN,* Sophia Palmer, agreed that financial ownership and editorial control must remain solely in the hands of nursing professionals. The journal committee first planned that individual nurses and alumnae would buy shares of stock in the new journal. Later, the ownership gradually shifted to the Associated Alumnae, newly renamed the American Nurses' Association (ANA). By 1912, with the exception of one stock ownership, the journal belonged to the ANA. Thus, "every nurse who was a member of any association affiliated with the American Nurses' Association was now equally an owner with every other nurse of this journal."[141] The *AJN* became the forum for debate and expression of nursing issues for members affiliated with the Associated Alumnae, the Superintendents' Society, and the American Federation of Nurses, and thus became "a necessary part of the trend in nursing progress."[142]

To assure nursing ownership of the journal, the founders established a journal stock company to publish the *AJN.* Individual nurses and alumnae associations initially purchased stock in the journal until the Associated Alumnae became financially able through a journal purchase fund to gradually buy out those stock owners who did not donate their holdings back to the Associated Alumnae. By 1910, the Associated Alumnae successfully reached its goal of sole ownership of the *AJN,* making professional control of the periodical an ". . . established fact."[143]

The *AJN* endeavored to educate and inform not only nurses but the public as well regarding developments in the newly-established and flourishing nursing profession. Its editors proposed to offer "the most progressive thought, and the latest news that the profession has to offer. . . ." As a general policy they encouraged the free flow of ideas on subjects of interest to professional nurses in both articles and reader response. Topics of interest in the journal often related to nursing education, nursing registration, woman suffrage, public health reforms, social reforms, and district, private duty, and hospital nursing. The editors welcomed all reader questions and opinions germane to nursing progress "fairly and without partisanship."[144] In order to maintain the journal's intended professional focus, the editors excluded those subjects that were considered personally malicious or which lacked broad interest for the profession. The journal was intended to advance professional education of the membership of the Associated Alumnae, the Superintendents' Society, and the National Organization for Public Health Nursing after it formed in 1912. The *AJN* also provided a link between the "workers and thinkers"[145] in nursing, offering a forum in which nursing educators, administrators, and trained nurses in all work settings could read about and respond to each other. Thus, the journal aimed to serve the interests of all trained nurses, and was instrumental in winning reforms in nurse registration and nursing education and training in the early twentieth century.

THE NATIONAL ASSOCIATION OF COLORED GRADUATE NURSES AND THE CONCERNS OF WOMEN OF COLOR IN THE NURSING PROFESSION

The history of the National Association of Colored Graduate Nurses (NACGN) paralleled that of the Superintendents' Society and the Associated Alumnae. The NACGN pursued similar goals for the professional development of nurses who were women of color. However, African-American nurses faced racially biased discriminatory practices which prohibited them from joining some state nursing associations, attending nurse training schools, sitting for the same state nurse registration exams (and in some states from even sitting for the exam), and from equal pay and employment opportunities with their white counterparts. As a result they formed a new professional organization to meet their needs in the profession. The NACGN was created in 1908 to overcome the unique problems American black women faced both as women and as trained nurses within the modern nursing movement. The NACGN battled the same issues as the Superintendents' Society and the Associated Alumnae: confronting opposition from the medical establishment, improving nursing education, bettering work conditions, and fighting for nursing registration, but had the additional burden of contending with racism within the nursing profession and society at large.[146]

The NACGN opened its membership to all black nurses, trained or untrained. However, there were distinct classifications to designate the educational backgrounds of its members: only registered nurses who graduated from a three-year training program were entitled to full membership; nurses who had not yet completed a training program joined as associate members; people interested in the advancement of nursing could join as lay members; and honorary memberships could be awarded by the NACGN board. NACGN membership grew from 125 nurses in 1912 to 500 nurses by 1920.[147]

The president of the NACGN, Adah Thoms, chronicled the history of the organization in her 1929 book, *Pathfinders, The Progress of Colored Graduate Nurses.* Martha Franklin was the organizer and founder of the NACGN. Beginning in 1906 and 1907, Franklin undertook a survey of African-American graduate nurses, superintendents of nurse training schools, and alumnae associations affiliated with African-American training schools to find out if there was sufficient interest in forming a professional nursing organization that would address issues confronting women of color in nursing. Because of segregation and prejudice, African-Americans were forced to develop a separate health care system after the Reconstruction Era. To accommodate their needs, an increasing number of hospitals and nurse training schools for African-Americans opened in America between the 1890s and 1920s. These segregated hospitals and schools provided medical and nursing care for the black population and provided the education for new physicians and nurses to serve that population. Franklin sent out two series of survey letters: in 1906 she sent more than 500 letters and, in 1907, she sent out more than 1,500.[148]

The Lincoln Hospital Alumnae Association, newly formed in 1903, responded favorably to Franklin's survey and agreed to organize a meeting of those nurses interested in a national organization. On August 25, 1908, in New York, the Lincoln Hospital Alumnae Association hosted the first meeting of the fledgling organization, which lasted for three days. Fifty-two nurses convened at St. Mark's Methodist Episcopal Church on 53rd Street in New York City to plan a new national organization. Martha Franklin presided at the first meeting, where many of the speeches addressed relevant topics in nursing such as the new and upcoming field of community health nursing.[149]

The November 1908 issue of the *AJN* included a report of the first NACGN convention. The *AJN* listed the papers presented at the conference as those given by physicians, titled "The Nurse Herself," "The

Demands for Nurses and Their Qualifications," and "Practical Points in Nursing," and papers by nurses which included, "Settlement Work in New York" given by Edith M. Carter, "Community Nursing on St. Helena's Island," by L. Viola Ford, and "District Nursing in London, England," by Mittie White from Augusta, Georgia. Additional papers delivered by nurses included titles such as "Private Nursing in Washington, D.C.," by Myntha C. Hankins, "Septicemia," by Mary E. Merrit of Leavenworth, Kansas, and "Is Trained Nursing a Necessity?" by Cora M. Garner, Kansas City, Kansas.[150]

At the meeting, a public health nurse from Henry Street Settlement House, Jane Hitchcock (1868–?), invited the NACGN members to visit the nearby Henry Street Nurses' Settlement the next day. On Friday, following the close of the first meeting, twenty-one NACGN members accepted Hitchcock's invitation and visited the nurses' settlement in New York City's lower east side. They heard Lillian Wald speak on the work of the settlement house, and Hitchcock gave them a tour of the dispensary, clubrooms, gymnasiums, and kindergarten sites organized in different homes in the community.[151]

On the final day of the conference, Thursday, August 27, 1908, the NACGN officially established itself as a professional organization and elected a slate of officers. C. Beatty of Lincoln Hospital installed the following elected officers: Martha Franklin from New Haven, Connecticut, as president; Viola V. Symons from Mt. Vernon, Ohio, as first vice-president; Edith M. Carter from New York City, as second vice-president; Mary F. Clarke from Richmond, Virginia, as recording secretary; L. Viola Ford from Charleston, South Carolina, as corresponding secretary; and Adah B. Samuels Thoms from New York, as treasurer. Before the conference adjourned, members at large selected a committee to develop the association's constitution and bylaws and set the next meeting of the NACGN for Boston on the last Tuesday in August, 1909. The *AJN* recorded that the NACGN members ended their first meeting, "all feeling that their higher ideal was accomplished."[152]

The NACGN held its first annual national convention in Boston in 1909 as planned. Its newly written constitution defined the goals of the NACGN: "to advance the standing and best interests of trained nurses, and to place the profession of nursing on the highest plane attainable."[153]

The NACGN's political activity centered around racial discrimination rather than sex discrimination. Between 1908 and 1952, the

NACGN addressed racially discriminating practices directed toward African-American nurses such as unfair state registration practices, unequal pay with white nurses, and unjust denial to serve the American Red Cross during both world wars.

From its inception the NACGN confronted prejudicial treatment of black nurses because of exclusionary state nurse registration legislation in some states. Although the Superintendents' Society and the Associated Alumnae campaigned for state nurse registration and licensure laws, these same laws in some southern states discriminated against trained nurses who were black. At their first meeting in August 1908, members passed a resolution that "all members of the Colored Graduate Nurses Association must be eligible to [sic] state registration."[154] The NACGN fought racial barriers in nursing as a collective and professional group. In their appeals to state legislators to enact nurse registration laws, African-American nurses had to contend with the same difficulties all women without the franchise faced in their political activist efforts. However, they had the additional burden of being black women in a political society dominated and controlled by white men. Thus, African-American nurses faced a double-edged sword of prejudice—as women and as blacks.

For most black women, racial discrimination at most nurse training schools throughout the country denied them the opportunity that Mary Mahoney (1848–1926), the first black trained nurse from the New England Hospital for Women and Children in Boston, had in 1879. Thus, to overcome racial prejudices affecting the education of African-American nurses and the provision of health care for African-Americans, separate nurse training schools and hospitals opened in the late nineteenth and early twentieth century.[155] In 1883, ten years after the opening of the first Nightingale training school in America, one of the first training schools for black women began at the MacVicar Hospital, connected with Spelman Seminary in Atlanta, Georgia.[156] Almost ten years later, in 1891, the Provident Hospital (1891–1966) in Chicago, under the supervision of Daniel H. Williams, a physician and superintendent of the hospital, opened a nurse training school for black women as well. In subsequent years, a series of nurse training schools for women of color opened: Hampton Institute in Virginia in 1891; Dixie Hospital in Virginia in 1891; John A. Andrew Hospital at Tuskegee Institute in 1892; Freedmen's Hospital in the District of Columbia in 1894; St.

Agnes Hospital in Raleigh, North Carolina, in 1895; the Frederick Douglass Memorial in Philadelphia in 1895; the Hospital and Training School for Nurses in Charleston, South Carolina, in 1896; the Flint-Goodridge Hospital in New Orleans in 1896; Lincoln Hospital and Home in New York City in 1898; the Mercy Hospital in Philadelphia in 1901; and Harlem Hospital School in New York City in 1923.[157]

By 1928, the thirty-six schools of nursing for women of color graduated almost 2,800 black nurses; the majority graduated from only ten of those schools.[158]

Documentation of the discriminatory patterns of accredited nurse training schools and the hiring practices of hospitals toward trained nurses of color appeared in the 1925 "Report on Informal Study of the Educational Facilities for Colored Nurses and Their Use in Hospital, Visiting, and Public Health Nursing." The Hospital Library and Service Bureau undertook this study, with funding from the Rockefeller Foundation, to learn which of the accredited nursing schools admitted black women and which of these hospitals hired black women. The data in this survey served as the background material used in a second Rockefeller-supported study known as "A Study of the Present Status of Negro Women in Nursing," directed by Ethel Johns.[159] Both studies gathered data on the employment pattern of African-American nurses in public health, private duty, and hospital nursing. The results clearly illustrated the discriminatory patterns trained black nurses faced in schools of nursing and in hiring practices. In the first study, of the 1,696 accredited schools included on a list prepared by the National League of Nursing Education (formally the Superintendents' Society and hereafter referred to as the NLNE), only 54 responded that they admitted black students while 1,588 responded they did not. Similarly black nurses faced limited employment opportunities: 66 hospitals used "colored graduate nurses," as compared to the 1,576 hospitals reported as not hiring black nurses on a regular basis. In public health, the odds were also stacked against nurses of color: 59 departments of health employed black nurses while 489 did not.[160]

Some comments gathered in the 1925 study also reveal the prejudicial treatment American black nurses experienced in their struggle to professionalize nursing. Alabama's former secretary of the state board of examiners, Miss H. McLean, reported that "colored students are admitted in training in the colored dept.'s but not all of the hospitals who admit colored patients have colored students. . . . No colored graduate nurses on duty in any hospitals which have not a colored dept."[161] Comments appeared in the study on the inferior training of black nurses, even from schools accredited by state boards. Miss B. W. McDonald, superintendent of the Public Health Nursing Association in Louisville, Kentucky, responded to the question, "Do you think colored nurses are preferable to white nurses for nursing among colored people?"[162] with the following: In theory, she thought that an interest by black nurses in caring for their own people should be encouraged. However, she could not see that black nurses served black communities better than their white counterparts. She justified her response by noting the vast difference in quality between the training of white and black nurses. "Even the best training for colored nurses hardly approximates the poorest training given to white nurses."[163]

McDonald concluded that service rendered by black nurses educated in such inferior schools "would necessarily be of lower grade"[164] than by graduate nurses of white schools. Although this sentiment was expressed in Kentucky, Kentucky was one of the twenty states in the union to have accredited schools of nursing for women of color. In 1925, twenty-seven states did not have any nurse training schools open to black women.[165]

The NACGN contended with racial intolerance while pioneering the development of the nursing profession. Fulfilling the resolution passed at the first meeting in August 1908, members of the NACGN continually worked for registration of all black graduate nurses and opposed the unfair "dual" registration laws being passed in some states. Since the first nurse registration law in North Carolina passed in 1903, in succeeding state licensure legislation, some states prohibited trained black nurses from taking registration examinations, or stipulated that separate exams be given to them.

Nurse registration acts were viewed by members of the Superintendents' Society, the Associated Alumnae, and the NACGN as a means of protecting the nursing profession and the public from untrained and poorly qualified practitioners and from inadequate schools of nursing. Between 1903 and 1914, forty states had organized state nurses associations and enacted permissive registration. Each state that passed such a law instituted a state board of examiners that monitored the criteria that determined which candidates qualified as registered nurses. The state board decided the acceptability of an applicant's preliminary education and developed the exam which tested an applicant's knowledge of nursing and regulated the licensure of registered nurses.[166]

African-American trained nurses struggled to be included among the trained nurses covered in each state's nurse registration law. The campaign of Ludie C. Andrews, a 1906 graduate of Spelman College nursing program and founder and superintendent of Grady Hospital Municipal Training School for Colored Nurses in Atlanta, exemplified the struggle to obtain state registration for black nurses. Andrews carried on a battle between 1910 to 1920 to guarantee the rights of black nurses to sit for the state nurse registration examination in Georgia.[167] During a discussion about nurse registration at the tenth annual meeting of the NACGN on August 21, 1917, Adah Thoms read a letter from Lucy Hale Topley, president of Spelman College in Atlanta, Georgia, to inform the NACGN that ". . . colored nurses were not recognized in the State of Georgia."[168] This discriminatory practice continued in Georgia until 1920, when African-American graduate nurses were granted the same rights of registration as white graduate nurses by the state board of examiners.[169]

The NACGN fought hard to redress the practice of exclusion of their members from some nursing registries and advocated the formation of a national registry specifically for African-American nurses working in private duty nursing. The NACGN recommended this registry in order to overcome overwhelming pay inequities that resulted from denied access to practice in white hospitals and the fewer job opportunities than their white counterparts in visiting nurse associations and health departments. When African-American trained nurses graduated they worked as private duty nurses in the homes of their patients because hospitals preferred to use pupil nurses, whether black or white, to provide service in the wards rather than hire the trained graduate. As private duty nurses, black as well as white graduates relied on case referrals for work; when registries barred them because of race, black graduate nurses found their livelihoods unduly threatened.[170]

Few jobs existed for black nurses trained in public health nursing, thus limiting the opportunities for employment other than private duty nursing. The hiring practices of public health departments and visiting nurse associations were studied in a survey conducted on the use of black nurses in public health nursing by Marjorie Stimson and Louise

Tattershall of the National Organization for Public Health Nursing (NOPHN) under the auspices of the Julius Rosenwald Fund. The NOPHN had studied this subject because of an "increasing amount of pubic health nursing conducted by and for Negroes." In a 1930 article in the journal, *Public Health Nurse,* Stanley Rayfield discussed the reports and statistics derived from that study which surveyed 97 public health agencies in eight northern cities including Chicago, New York, Detroit, Cincinnati, Cleveland, Philadelphia, St. Louis, and Dayton.[171]

The findings displayed the restricted hiring practices of health departments and visiting nurse associations which hired too few black nurses in comparison with the black population they served. The black public health nurses surveyed in the study had public health experience mostly in urban settings: only 3 out of 231 nurses had previous rural or southern public health nursing experience. In one city where too few black public health nurses were employed, Rayfield found "that the health department employed a staff only .9 percent Negro although 65 percent of its cases are Negro."[172]

By 1917, to counteract the restricted hiring practices of black graduate nurses in hospitals, public health nursing, and in private duty nursing, Adah Thoms urged the National Association of Colored Graduate Nurses to establish a national registry for black nurses. The unpublished minutes of the NACGN recorded the formation of a national registry committee at the tenth annual meeting of the NACGN in August 1917. While the unpublished minutes of the NACGN did not furnish details of the committee's work, Adah Thoms reported at the eleventh annual meeting of August 20, 1918, that the national registry had provided work for twelve nurses.[173]

Since its beginning in 1908, the NACGN addressed the disparity in pay between its members and their white nurse counterparts. Unlike the other two professional organizations, the Superintendents' Society and the Associated Alumnae, which argued for pay equity with men, the NACGN first had to fight the battle for pay equity against pervasive racial discrimination. As a result, this issue was frequently referred to at NACGN meetings. For example, a graduate of Tuskegee Institute training school and later president of the NACGN from 1923–1926, Petra Pinn, reported at the executive board meeting of December 3, 1918, that some states objected to paying "colored" nurses the same as white nurses. As the same meeting, Adah Thoms argued that the same standards of remuneration be set for registered nurses regardless of race.[174]

Nurses of color faced racial barriers not only in civilian practice but in the military setting as well. Since its inception, the NACGN worked towards confronting racial restraints that prohibited trained black nurses from serving during World War I. As America entered World War I in 1917, the racist policy of the American Red Cross barred entrance of African-American nurses who wanted to volunteer. Exclusion also blocked their acceptance into the United States Army Nurse Corps because entrance to the corps required referral from the American Red Cross Nursing Service.[175] Believing in her members' right to serve, NACGN president Adah Thoms argued this point at association meetings and in numerous correspondences with Jane Delano (1858 [1862?]–1919), organizer of the American Red Cross Nursing Service and former president of the Associated Alumnae (1909–1911). As professional women, NACGN members wanted to serve their nation. However, when members were denied the opportunity to serve abroad as Red Cross nurses, the NACGN members expressed their patriotism and loyalty by reporting the number of individual black nurses who subscribed to the Liberty Loans being sold. They felt that ". . . the public should see what we have done and [still] to be ignored professionally."[176]

With a membership that had now grown to 500 members, the NACGN was outraged that qualified black nurses were barred from service because of race while there existed great shortages of trained nurses at home and abroad during the war years. While at the eleventh annual NACGN meeting of August 20, 1918, held in St. Louis, Missouri, a representative of the medical society in St. Louis, Missouri, a Dr. Curtis, commented on the omission of military service by black nurses during the war. Curtis said that while Americans fought the Germans abroad, pioneer African-American nurses fought prejudice here at home. With this sentiment in mind, Thoms opened the conference requesting that black nurses be sent to Europe to serve.[177]

At the Wednesday, August 21, morning session of the eleventh annual convention of the NACGN, members heard greetings from Jane Delano read to them. Delano, responding to the concern of the NACGN members that nurses of color were not able to volunteer their services to the American Red Cross during the war, stated that the American Red Cross was "blameless for the colored nurses not having been utilized" in the war.[178] Delano, who supported the use of NACGN members for overseas duty in the Red Cross, explained that the surgeon-general of the army enforced the army's policy that restricted the number of black nurses selected. As a result of this policy, the surgeon-general had refused to authorize acceptance of African-American nurses into the Red Cross. This policy remained in effect until, overwhelmed by the civilian registered nurse shortages and the devastating effects of the influenza epidemic (1917–1918), African-American nurses were permitted to enter the American Red Cross Nursing Service in July 1918.

Finally, in December 1918, following acceptance into the American Red Cross Nursing Service, eighteen black nurses entered the Army Nurse Corps. These women sent a letter to their colleagues at the 1919 twelfth annual convention of the NACGN in Boston describing the first half-year of their work and the obstacles to be overcome; they wrote that "as colored women and nurses . . . [they had to be] . . . firm, tactful, earnest, cheerful and observant . . ." and that they prayed for their success.[179]

The NACGN hoped to integrate the American Red Cross with their members when they saw the increasing shortage of nurses arise because of World War I and the 1917 influenza epidemic. However, unsuccessful in securing military work for many of its membership, the NACGN looked to other avenues for serving African-American military men. Adah Thoms guided the association's participation in the newly established Circle for Negro War Relief in November 1917. Similar in purpose to the American Red Cross, the circle offered relief services to black military men and their families in this country and abroad. Thoms organized the Blue Circle Nurses which included black public health nurses who were hired by the Circle of Negro War Relief to care for the families of disabled servicemen at home. Following the war, the Circle for Negro War Relief renamed itself the Circle for Negro Relief and focused its work on providing public health nursing and education to rural black communities in the South.[180]

One African-American woman who successfully joined the American Red Cross in 1917, Frances Elliot Davis (1882–1965), was a 1913 graduate of the Freedmen's Hospital in Washington, D.C. Davis applied to the American Red Cross after working for three years as a private duty nurse in the Washington area. As part of her admission into the

Red Cross, Davis had to complete the Town and Country Nursing Service Course, a one-year course in rural public health nursing sponsored by the American Red Cross and given at Teachers College, Columbia University. The Red Cross advanced Davis $500 to pay for the cost of the additional preparation. While in the program at Teachers College, Davis listened to the lectures of prominent nursing educator Adelaide Nutting and gained practical experience under the auspices of Lillian Wald at the Henry Street Settlement in New York. Davis became the first black woman to enter the Town and Country Course and she became the first black nurse accepted into the American Red Cross. However, in spite of her success in the training period and in providing nursing service in the Town and Country Nursing Service in Jackson, Tennessee, the American Red Cross denied Davis's application to serve overseas during World War I; trained black nurses were not accepted into the Army Nurse Corps until World War II (1941–1945).[181]

The NACGN shared with other professional nursing associations an interest in the issues that pertained to the advancement of the nursing profession in America. Besides the NLNE and the Associated Alumnae (hereafter called the ANA) these associations included the National Organization for Public Health Nursing (NOPHN), which formed in 1912. Unlike the NLNE and the ANA, the NOPHN allowed individuals to join the organization, thus enabling membership for trained black nurses. The public health movement which swept America at the beginning of the twentieth century created the new field in public health nursing and a new organization called the NOPHN; black trained black nurses found work in this area and acceptance into the NOPHN as well.[182]

From its inception in 1908, the National Association of Colored Graduate Nurses maintained a working relationship with Lillian Wald, public health nurse and founder of the Henry Street Settlement. Wald and the leaders of the NACGN had a shared mission to improve the health of all citizens living in both rural and urban centers. Black public health nurses most often worked in black communities in which a nurse's daily work might include sanitary health teaching, newborn baby care, and care of the sick at home; however, their job was more difficult because black public health nurses confronted higher mortality rates, higher levels of poverty, and fewer health care facilities to serve their constituents than their white counterparts.[183] The issues of public health nursing thus provided a vital connection between the two groups which affected the history of both the NACGN and the NOPHN.

Throughout its existence between 1908 and 1951, the NACGN had to contend with America's biased treatment of black Americans. Similarly, in the profession of nursing, all four nursing organizations, the NLNE, the ANA, the NACGN, and the NOPHN had to overcome the results of such racism. Two years before the founding of the National Association of Colored Graduate Nurses, activist Lavinia Dock, while at the thirteenth annual convention in August 1910, spoke out against prejudicial treatment of any professional nurse; she cited the need for practical ethics to be demonstrated in nursing and ardently hoped that the nursing association [the ANA] would never "get to the point where it draws the color line against our negro sister nurses." Dock feared that the tremendous growth of the ANA would lead to a change in the treatment of nurses of color. She had always believed that the nurse association was one place in America where color boundaries were not drawn. However, as the association expanded throughout the country, Dock witnessed "evidences" that made her think "that this cruel and unchristian and unethical prejudice might creep in here in our association."[184] Dock said that under no circumstances should nurses emulate the cruel prejudices displayed by men, and concluded her remarks by urging nurses to treat each nurse of color "as we would like to be treated ourselves."[185]

The NACGN worked consistently between 1908 and 1951 to break down discriminatory practices in education, practice, and organizational activities.[186] During these years, the NACGN periodically sent representatives to the other nursing organizations as a way of combating discriminatory practices. On August 17, 1920, during the thirteenth annual meeting of the NACGN in Tuskegee, Alabama, President Adah Thoms explained why she had previously asked that a representative from the NACGN attend the meetings of the white nurse associations, specifically the ANA. Thoms wanted to establish this contact because she believed that black nurses were being discussed at ANA meetings.[187] Petra Pinn had been the selected representative and had attended the ANA's annual meeting the previous April in Atlanta, Georgia. Pinn reported back to the NACGN at the August meeting that she had heard some disparaging remarks made during a presentation comparing white nurses with colored nurses. Although the minutes did not include further discussion, it was agreed that NACGN should attend the three other nursing organizations.[188]

Whenever asked, the NACGN responded to surveys about the organization from the other nursing organizations. During the 1920 convention in Tuskegee, Thoms gave the NACGN a copy of the questionnaire, "How the Problem of Training Colored Nurses Can Be Met In the South," sent to her by the National Program Committee of the ANA, the NLNE, and the NOPHN. Adah Thoms reported that she had completed the survey and had ". . . expressed herself freely."[189]

The sharing of information and representation contributed to the eventual integration of the NACGN with the other three nursing organizations. The NACGN had tackled a series of important issues between its founding in 1908 and its integration with the ANA in 1951; problems related to inadequately supported nurse training schools, unequal remuneration, separate and unequal nurse training schools, inadequate primary and secondary schools which impacted on adequate preparation of future candidates in nurse training, and token or infrequent representation of black nurses in leadership positions. In spite of working alone towards professional goals, the leadership of the NACGN sought integration into the other nursing professional groups. In 1948, after a long battle against racism, an NACGN recommendation to the ANA to form an intergroup relations program was adopted. The intergroup relations program formed to facilitate the eventual integration of black nurses into the profession of nursing. To meet this goal, the intergroup relations program began programs which developed leadership skills of black nurses, facilitated improved program development in state and local nursing associations, and removed racial discrimination in all occupational settings in nursing.[190]

Patterns of integration in American nursing changed following World War II. Until the war, only 42 nursing schools out of 1,200 schools accepted black candidates and 28 of those schools admitted black students only; none of the armed services included a black nurse among its staff, but by 1942, 56 African-American nurses were inducted into the army and by the end of the war there were more than 500. Two thousand black women enrolled in the U.S. Army Nurses Corps as a result of the 1943 passage of the Nurses Training Act, known as the Bolton Act because of the work of Frances Payne Bolton (1885–1977), congresswoman from Ohio and friend of nursing and the

NACGN. Bolton was instrumental in passing this legislation, which provided free nurse education in a thirty-month course in return for which nurses pledged military or critical civilian service.[191]

While the racism experienced by black nurses continued following World War II, the ANA, and the NLNE took steps to open their doors to African-American registered nurses. Following the success of the National Organization for Public Health Nursing, these organizations changed to a policy which allowed individual memberships, circumventing state regulations that prohibited African-Americans from state associations, hence, the national organization. The ANA house of delegates at their 1950 convention passed a resolution that emphasized the rights of participation of minority members within the ANA and called for the elimination of discrimination in practice settings. On January 26, 1951, members of the NACGN voted to dissolve their own organization and transfer its members into the ANA. The Intergroup Relations Committee established in 1948 directed the association's new policies and facilitated integration of its new members.[192]

Former executive secretary of the NACGN and activist in the integration of black nursing in America, Mabel Staupers (1890–1990), firmly believed that the dissolution of the NACGN, forty-two years after it had been founded, would lead to an integrated nursing world in America. She believed that nursing served the "cause of health,"[193] and since health and disease were not subject to racial barriers, nurses could work together "to the end that this world of ours may become increasingly better."[194]

NATIONAL ORGANIZATION FOR PUBLIC HEALTH NURSING

Responding to the needs of the newly emerging specialization of public health nurse, the National Organization for Public Health Nursing (NOPHN) formed on June 7, 1912. The role of the public health nurse had expanded as a direct result of America's public health movement of the nineteenth and twentieth centuries. As urban centers faced dirty streets, overcrowded tenement houses, and poor ventilation in homes, this new movement earned the attention of the public and government.[195] American trained nurses became the new public health nurses as they visited patients in homes, factories, and schools. They worked in ethnically, racially, and religiously diverse communities, nursing the sick and teaching the well proper sanitary health care behaviors.[196]

During the Progressive Era, the public's health became an important concern of social reformers. Reformers applied their activism to improving sanitary conditions in cities and in the countryside and set their goals on such issues as attaining pure water and a clean milk supply for the public. Because of the widely spreading interest in improving sanitary conditions of local municipalities, graduate nurses found a new professional setting in which to work that differed from that of the hospital or private duty. Trained nurses who mostly had worked as private duty nurses or in supervisory roles in hospitals, now worked as pubic health nurses in the community. Away from the employment by hospitals or wealthy private duty patients, the public health nurse worked in visiting nurse services, public health agencies, large insurance companies, boards of education, and industrial companies.[197]

One public health nurse described the difference between the work of public health nursing and private duty as "one is living and the latter is existing."[198] A public health nurse from Washington wrote that she preferred public health nursing after twenty years of private duty nursing because it offered a "wider scope"[199] for her "personal tastes, a more independent life, a life more free from restraint . . ."[200] More importantly, public health nurses no longer had to be kept guessing whether they would be called to work on a case "today, tomorrow, or next week. . . ."[201] Most public health nurses responded favorably to the freedom that this new practice setting offered, citing as examples the regular hours and pay, increased possibilities for promotion and advancement, and the variety of interesting experiences. This new setting offered nurses "movement, initiative, getting out in the open, regular salary, eight hours of intensive and interesting work, [and] time for one's friends . . . ."[202] Whereas private duty nurses remained in the home twenty-four hours a day with one patient or case until they were no longer needed, the public health nurse visited a number of cases each day and lived outside of the patient's home. More importantly, the public health nurse refocused nursing care away from treatment and care of the sick to include health teaching about proper hygiene, disease prevention, and health promotion in the community. This aspect of public health nurse work was highly valued. As explained by one public health nurse, "prevention of disease seems to be preferred to the curative phase of the work."[203]

Public health nurses emphasized an agenda of prevention as well as treatment of disease. They connected their health teaching with the prevention of such diseases as syphilis, gonorrhea, tuberculosis, childhood diseases, and "so-called chronic conditions . . . ."[204] These nurses had to be a "middleman of science"[205] and carry the message of personal and public health into the home, the factory, the school, or wherever people could be reached.

The public health nurse responded to the changing health needs of American society, which experienced in the twentieth century greater degrees of industrialization, urbanization, and immigration. These social changes presented an ever increasing number of health-related problems because of communicable diseases, malnutrition, overcrowded housing, discrimination among different groups, and exploitation of workers. These factors influenced those active in the public health movement to find ways to improve the health conditions they encountered. Public health professionals combined nineteenth-century sanitary reforms with the application of the bacteriological discoveries in disease prevention such as those found for tuberculosis and smallpox.[206] The public health nurse carried the message of public health out into the community as exemplified by the work of the early visiting nurse associations and Philanthropic agencies of the late 1880s, which provided home nursing services to the sick poor in America.[207] These public health nurses taught the "elementary laws of healthful living,"[208] and preventative health care among families in communities, workers in factories, and children in schools.

One of the most influential public health agencies at the end of the nineteenth and beginning of the twentieth century was that of the Henry Street Nurses Settlement, founded by Lillian Wald and Mary Brewster in 1893. Both graduates from New York Hospital Training school in 1891, Wald and Brewster demonstrated the importance and directed the development of public health and visiting nurse services throughout the country and the world.

Wald wrote that during her first twenty years at Henry Street, she experienced a particular awakening of social concerns in America. For example, people began to show an interest in protecting the health and welfare of children and began to shoulder the social responsibilities required to make a change. To explain this development, Wald singled out the women's experience, because women in particular had experienced a greater awakening of these social responsibilities ". . . since the period coincides with their freer admission to public and professional life."[209] A visiting nurse who lived at Henry Street experienced an opportunity not only to work as a nurse, but also to live with different people and experience new ideas that she would be unable to find at other "more fixed and older institutions."[210] Influenced by Lillian Wald, the nurses at Henry Street related all social, economic, and industrial conditions to the health and well-being of the patients they served. As a result, public health nursing earned a reputation of activism during the Progressive Era in America between the 1880s and World War I, and Wald earned the distinction of being one of the most well-known women of the progressive generation.[211]

The activities of Henry Street attracted nursing activists such as Lavinia Dock to settlement house work. Dock had described herself as a "free-lance" in nursing until she finally "reached the Henry Street Settlement with Miss Wald."[212] In 1896, three years following the opening of the settlement house, Dock, at the age of 38, joined the nurses at Henry Street. While living at Henry Street, Dock said she began to understand "social systems"[213] and saw "the processes of evolution in human society . . ." which became clearer to her the more she read, was told or saw, "the downtrodden, miserable existence of the world's workers." This she said gave her "the revolutionary coloring" which had become a "definite" part of her.[214] Profoundly influenced by her experiences at Henry Street, Dock settled among these social reformers for twenty years.

Dock describes the daily routine of the nurses living together at the Henry Street Settlement. She wrote that in a typical day, the nurses at their breakfast together at half past seven giving themselves an opportunity to read their mail and plan their day. After the rooms were "set in order" and the new cases distributed among the nurses, the nurses set out into the community to care for the sick. The nurses worked independently, each managing her time according to her own case load of clients and calling in the physician only when necessary. The nurses returned to the settlement house for luncheon where, Dock explained, they usually found some "visitor or visitors interested and interesting, for no dull or stupid people ever appear at the Settlement."[215] Following lunch, the nurse completed their afternoon nursing visits and returned to the settlement to begin the health classes they offered to the families in the community. Dock described a class given to foreign born mothers in "simple home nursing and hygiene" by one nurse who spoke Yiddish. Another nurse offered cooking classes and demonstrated how to prepare well-cooked food "from the least expensive materials." For the girls fourteen and fifteen years of age, the settlement nurses organized a club for them to come and learn simple skills in housework, hygiene, care of the sick, cooking, and physical culture. Dock wrote that the nurses also acted as "older sister and adviser" to these young girls.[216]

Influenced by its English counterpart, which was called district nursing, public health nursing evolved in America between the late 1800s and early 1900s. Many of these earlier services had religious affiliations and required nurses to provide nursing care for the sick poor while being alert to the patients' religious needs as well. Prior to the existence of the Henry Street Settlement, the New York City Mission, a religion-based service, used trained nurses to visit the city's sick poor in 1877. Two years later, in 1879, the Ethical Culture Society, a nonsecular religious group, established visiting nursing services to the sick poor. The Ethical Culture nurses worked with the free medical services offered at existing dispensaries. During the same period a series of autonomous visiting nurse associations emerged, including the Buffalo District Nursing Association in 1885, the Boston Instructive District Visiting Nurse Association in 1886, Visiting Nurses Association of Philadelphia in 1886, and the Chicago Visiting Nurse Association in 1889.[217]

Despite the existence of these and other visiting nurse associations prior to the founding of the Henry Street Settlement in New York City in 1893, the New York settlement exerted tremendous influence on the visiting nurse associations that formed after 1893. The Henry Street Settlement offered visiting nursing services to the community and provided a communal life for the nurses living at the settlement house. At Henry Street the nurses lived in the community they served and thus experienced firsthand the social, cultural, economic, and political problems specific to community residents.

Both Wald and Brewster had envisioned a new visiting nurse service that did not rely on any religious affiliation or have any connection to free dispensary service or to a single physician as was the case with the nursing services available in New York City at the time. In order to create a public health nursing service that considered "the dignity and independence of the patients,"[218] she charged a small fee for nursing services to be determined by a patient's ability to pay. Moreover, the settlement's visiting nurses would respond to referrals from all people, not only physicians, thereby permitting neighbors and family members to directly contract for needed nursing services. Referrals would be accepted from several physicians rather than from only one as was the typical practice of the private duty nurse. As a result of these innovative ideas, Wald believed that the Henry Street visiting nurses philosophically changed the relationship between patient and nurse; a visit by a Henry Street Settlement nurse signaled to neighbors that the family could provide needed care for a sick member rather than feeling "chagrin at having the neighbors see in her an agent whose presence proclaimed the family's poverty . . . ."[219]

Wald's visionary leadership extended into the education of future public health nurses. Attentive to what the trained nurse needed to learn about public health and the concomitant political, social, and economic issues, Wald in 1914 designed a course in public health nursing to be offered as one of the post-graduate courses at Teachers College at Columbia University. Students who enrolled in the course were already trained graduate nurses who needed additional education in order to adequately fulfill the required role of the public health nurse. Henry Street and later satellites of the settlement house provided the field work for the course and many of the settlement house nurses taught the students. In addition, the course at Teachers College assisted other schools to model similar courses in their curriculum.[220]

By 1902, following an experiment Wald designed which demonstrated the importance of using public health nurses in public schools, nurses for the first time were hired by local municipalities, marking an "extraordinary development of the public control of the physical condition of children."[222] During Wald's one-month experiment, which she carried out in four New York City public schools, public health nurses placed in each school showed that with proper and immediate treatment of some contagious diseases and with instruction on proper sanitary behaviors, students missed fewer classes.[222]

While issues of public health piqued America's interest, public health nurses demonstrated their vast usefulness in this area. Between 1894 and 1905, America witnessed the rapid growth of 171 visiting nurse associations in an estimated 110 cities and towns which employed more than 455 nurses.[223] Often, local women's clubs and societies raised money to support the work of a public health nurse in a community. The public appreciated nursing's efforts in caring for the sick, in disease prevention, and health promotion, hence, public health nurses found themselves hired by "states and municipalities, churches, manufacturing and commercial firms and industries."[224]

Public health nursing exerted a major influence on the development of public health in America which was rarely recorded.[225] Wald reported that the importance of public health nurses could not be "overestimated" and informed the public of the vast increase in public health nurses from 1,413 in 1909 to 15,865 in 1933.[226] Philanthropic visiting nurses associations grew from 500 in 1909 to more than 1,000 by 1926.[227] Public health nurses had demonstrated that the success in their work further justified a continued increase in their numbers.[228]

The public health nurses at Henry Street found that their nursing treatments administered to sick infants and children in the home greatly increased the survival rate of young persons as compared to similar treatments in four New York City hospitals. Wald asserted that the 1914 records at Henry Street had demonstrated that their nursing staff had cared for 3,535 cases of pneumonia of all ages; these cases yielded a mortality rate of 8.05 percent, which compared favorably to the 1,612 cases of pneumonia treated at four large cosmopolitan hospitals, which yielded a mortality rate of 31.2 percent. Among children under two years of age, the mortality rate for pneumonia in the home was 9.3 percent, while one of the four hospitals had a mortality rate of 51 percent. The rate of the four hospitals combined was 38 percent. According to Wald, home nursing meant that children who had recovered from pneumonia had not been exposed to cross infection at home, as at a hospital; in addition, whole families benefited from the home health teaching of the public health nurses. Clearly, such documentation supported the drive already underway by nursing leaders to increase the numbers of public health nurses in the community.[229]

By 1912, public health nursing had experienced rapid growth and attracted great community interest. However, there was no organization that monitored the professional growth of nursing within the new public health movement. Although many small visiting nurse associations existed that hired and assisted the new public health nurse in her work, many nursing leaders felt that these association sometimes lacked knowledge of the "fundamental requirements" needed for visiting nursing.[230] The increasing presence of nurses insufficiently trained in home care and improperly supervised by inadequately trained managers, mobilized the leaders of public health nursing. Influential spokeswomen such as Lillian Wald, Mary Gardner, Mary Brewster, and Lavinia Dock advocated a new national nursing organization to address the issues of the visiting nurse and they found that the leadership of both the Superintendents' Society and the ANA supported the formation of a fourth nursing organization. In January 1912, a joint committee was appointed by the Superintendents' Society [NLNE] and the ANA to ". . . determine some method of standardization for visiting nurse work."[231]

Lillian Wald chaired this committee, whose members included Jane Delano; Ella Phillips Crandall (1871–1938), supervisor at Henry Street and executive secretary of the National Organization for Public Health Nursing (NOPHN); Edna Louise Foley (1879–1943), superintendent of the Chicago Visiting Nurse Association and advocate for the rights of black nurses; Mary Beard (1876–1946), superintendent of the Instructive District Nursing Association; Mary Gardner; and a Miss Kerr. After several meetings this committee reported back to the Superintendents' Society [NLNE] and the ANA in the summer of 1912, at the fifteenth annual convention of the ANA, that a great need for standardization of visiting nurse work existed and the time was ". . . ripe for the formation of a national visiting nurse association."[232]

Prior to its report the joint committee had written to more than 1,000 organizations that employed visiting and public health nurses. Its letter invited each society or association to send delegates to a 9 a.m. meeting at the Auditorium Hotel on Wednesday, June 5, 1912, during the ANA's fifteenth annual convention in Chicago. The delegates sent would help establish an organization for public health nursing which would have the "power to render valuable assistance and guidance to public spirited citizens, and to nurses who wish to share in the great campaign for public health."[233]

Public health nurses throughout the country responded favorably to the joint committee's invitation; delegates from sixty-nine organizations attended the June meeting in Chicago. Another twenty-nine agencies wrote to the joint committee that they supported the planning meeting for the new organization but could not send delegates due to financial constraints.[234] At the meeting, delegates mapped out plans for the new national association for public health nurses. Both the Superintendents' Society and the ANA approved the plans for the new organization and the chair of the joint committee, Mary Gardner, reflected that such collective action of the two established nursing associations made "for the first time one strong, united body of nurses."[235]

Delegates carefully debated the name of their new organization to assure deriving one that reflected the variety of public health nursing settings found in schools, factories, welfare agencies, tuberculosis clinics, and social services. The delegates preferred the term public health nurse rather than that of visiting nurse, to include all nurses involved in public health nursing. In addition, the newly-constituted membership elected to use the term "nursing" rather than "nurses" in the organization's title, which would permit the inclusion of all people interested in expanding the field of public health. Thus, one of the unique qualities of the National Organization for Public Health Nursing was reflected in its name—that its membership was extended to all who worked towards public health education and service, including "lay workers with nurses."[236]

The charter members of the new association defined their goals in the National Organization for Public Health Nursing constitution: to stimulate knowledge in public health, to facilitate harmonious relations among the workers and supporters in public health, to develop standards of ethics and techniques, and to act as a clearing house for those interested in public health work. The constitution provided for three classifications of membership. Any organization engaged in public health nursing, such as those run by private societies, churches, business enterprises, cities, state boards, or any governmental body, could become a corporate member and would be permitted to send to the National Organization for Public Health Nursing meetings one nurse, who was a member of the ANA, as their voting delegate. Any nurse engaged in public health nursing who was a member of the ANA was eligible to be an individual member and thus hold voting privileges. The charter members included an associate member category to assure that the NOPHN represented all segments of public health workers, including any individual not a nurse, as well as those nurses who did not work in public health and/or were ineligible for individual membership. Associate members were accorded all the rights of membership except the right to vote at meetings. All members could speak and participate at NOPHN meetings and receive literature sent from the organization. However, voting rights in all categories remained in the hands of registered nurses who were members of the ANA.

Membership dues financially supported the work of the NOPHN and were kept "purposefully low" so that "no nurse nor society interested in public health nursing need be excluded."[237] Corporate members paid $10 a year, individual members paid $1 a year, and the associate members paid $3 a year. A NOPHN pamphlet published during the organization's third year listed a third fee of $25 a year for sustaining membership. Between 1913 and 1914, membership in the NOPHN increased from 587 to 1,305.[238]

Activities of the NOPHN included: conducting studies on the various associations involved in public health nursing; publishing *Public Health Nurse Quarterly* and two bulletins a year; adopting a standard record card; and maintaining a central office, an executive, and a traveling secretary. The main purpose was to help public health nurses learn the professional role in the community by providing information, setting standards, developing advanced courses, finding jobs, and advising them when needed. The organization supported the standardization and coordination of the 1,346 public and private public health organizations, and in addition, provided "reliable morbidity statistics" to the public as a result of adopting a uniform standard record card in which to collect these statistics.[239]

PROFESSIONAL ORGANIZATIONS FIND THEIR POLITICAL VOICE

Spearheaded by the NLNE and the ANA, the National Organization for Public Health Nursing constituted a strong coalition of trained nurses that advanced the nursing profession. Meetings among the three groups supported each other's efforts to advance and improve nursing in America. While president of the NLNE from 1913 to 1918, Clara Noyes (1869–1936) acknowledged the close ties and shared responses expressed by the three organizations towards the socio–economic and political climate of the Progressive Era. Through their collective activism in nursing, these women improved the conditions within their profession as well as improved the lives of the patients and families that they met in their practice in hospitals, schools, industries, and communities.

Their feminist activities could be seen through the political use of their organizations to alter society's attitudes toward nursing, women's work and education, and public health. These nurses attempted to improve the image society held of nurses to that of professional women so as to attract new recruits into the field. Whether avidly feminist or not, nursing leaders, like other women in the woman's movement, organized their nursing constituency into national associations so that they could control their practice and education. Once organized, these nursing leaders influenced and changed the public's ideas about nursing and health care. Recognizing the feminist strength of these nursing leaders at the fifteenth annual convention of the ANA in 1912, Sophia Palmer praised nursing for producing the *AJN,* which she considered the best women's magazine ever published. Palmer asked, "Where is there another journal owned and edited and managed by women that is anything more than a little newspaper?" and commented that she thought the *AJN* was "the greatest journal that any group of women have ever put forth."[240] The contents of each issue of the journal represented the practical work of women in nursing whose creativity, knowledge, energy, and finances formed this nursing journal, and hence modeled American nursing at the beginning of the twentieth century.

Each of the four nursing organizations, the American Nurses' Association, the National League of Nursing Education, the National Association of Colored Graduate Nurses, and the National Organization for Public Health Nursing, nurtured the growth of the nursing profession. They built coalitions of nurses who worked toward improving and standardizing nursing education, accrediting schools, and defining their practice. While all four organizations worked at establishing and elevating standards of the whole profession, each association retained its specific interests and members.

The woman's movement remained an underlying theme throughout each group's formation and years of growth. Professional graduate nurses recognized the unique position they maintained in American society as a collective force of women engaged in professional activities. Through their organizations they sought control of their profession by developing standards of practice, educational requirements, and state registration laws. Organized in their professional associations, nurses created a strong voice to argue with the opposition for the control they sought. They had to challenge physicians who wanted compliant nurses to fill their medical orders and to retain a handmaiden relationship with them. As a result of medical opposition, nurse licensure laws were slow to be enacted nationwide because of these strong political opponents, thus requiring extraordinary political agitation by the state nursing associations formed for that very purpose.[241]

As nurses in their associations politically struggled to obtain state licensure, the inability to vote for such a change epitomized the meaning of woman suffrage. Consequently, the professional work of each organization fused nursing's singleness of purpose with other woman's rights advocates. Nurses shared the belief of those in the suffrage movement that the vote would ensure women's rights in the home and the workplace, thus the franchise came to symbolize personal and professional freedom.

NOTES

1. Sophia Palmer, Training School Alumnae Associations. *First and Second Annual Conventions of the ASSTSN* (Harrisburg, PA: Harrisburg Publishing, 1897), 55. ANHNC, TC-CU, MML, New York; Reverby, *Annual Conventions,* 55.

2. Dock and Stewart, *A Short History,* 158.

3. Kalisch and Kalisch, *The Advance of American Nursing,* 144–5.

4. Stewart, *The Education of Nurses,* 93–95, for a description of the opposition to nursing education and the dual function of the training school, and Report of the Committee for the Study of Nursing Education, *Nursing and Nursing Education in the United States* (1923, reprint New York: Garland Publishing Company, 1984), 194–5.

5. Louise Darche, "Employments for Women, No. 2, Trained Nursing" *The Delineator: A Journal of Fashion, Culture and Fine Arts,* 82 (June 1894); 667–668; Victor Robinson, *White Caps: The Story of Nursing* (Philadelphia: Lippincott, 1946), 304; Dorothy Tao, "Louise M. Darche," Bullough, Sentz, and Stein, *American Nursing* 2: 75–77.

6. Burgess, *Nurses, Patients, and Pocketbooks,* 250, 258, 266–270. In a 1928 study by the graduating committee, 54 percent of all nurses practicing were private duty nurses; Dock and Stewart, *A Short History of Nursing,* 159–160; Reverby, "The Search for the Hospital Yardstick: Nursing

and the Rationalization of Hospital Work," 207; Susan Reverby, "Reforming the Hospital Nurse: The Management of American Nursing," in *The Sociology of Health and Illness: Critical Perspectives,* eds. Peter Conrad and Rochelle Kern (New York: St. Martin's Press), 211–223; Strauss, "The Structure and Ideology of American Nursing: An Interpretation," 70–71.

7. W. Gilman Thompson, *Training Schools for Nurses,* (New York: Putnam's, 1883), quoted in Stewart, *The Education of Nurses,* 94.

8. W. Gilman Thompson, "The Overtrained Nurse," *New York Medical Journal* (April 28, 1908) in Kalisch and Kalisch, *The Advance of American Nursing,* 185.

9. Stewart, *The Education of Nurses,* 93–99 and 107–8, for a general discussion of the opinion of hospital boards and physicians regarding professional nursing education; Kalisch and Kalisch, *The Advance of American Nursing,* 144–145 and 150–53, for general discussion of medical opposition regarding nursing education and a chart which compares entrance requirements, texts, and fees paid to students and instructors at five nurse training schools between 1873 and 1878; Franklin North, "A New Profession for Women," 39, for initial medical opposition to the opening of nurse training at Bellevue.

10. Appendix A. Graduation diploma from Boston City Hospital Training School, 1897.

11. Dock and Stewart, *A Short History of Nursing,* 285–287; Susan Reverby, "'Neither for the Drawing Room nor for the Kitchen': Private Duty Nursing in Boston, 1873–1920," in *Women and Health in America: Historical Readings,* ed. Judith Walzer Leavitt (Madison, WI: University of Wisconsin Press, 1984), 454–466, for a discussion of private duty nursing and the ambiguous social position they faced while working in a patient's home.

12. Lavinia Dock, "A National Association for Nurses and Its Legal Organization," *Proceedings of the Third Annual Convention of the ASSTSN* (Harrisburg, PA: Harrisburg Publishing, 1896), 47–48; reprinted in Susan Reverby, ed., *Annual Convention 1893–1899 ASSTSN* (New York: Garland Publishing Company, 1985), 47–48; reprinted in Birnbach and Lewenson, *First Words,* 303, for a general discussion about how the Woman's Christian Temperance Union, the General Federation of Women's Clubs, and the Association of Collegiate Alumnae unite their members.

13. Irwin, *Angels and Amazons,* 443–499, for brief histories of women's organizations which formed during the late nineteenth and early twentieth centuries; Mary Cadwalder Jones, "Women's Opportunities in Town and

Country," in *The Woman's Book Dealing Practically With the Modern Conditions of Home-Life, Self-Support, Education, Opportunities, and Every-Day Problems.* 2 vols. (New York: Scribner's Sons, 1894), II: 188–91; Elizabeth M. Jamieson and Mary F. Sewall, *Trends in Nursing History: Their Relationships to World Events,* 4th ed. (Philadelphia: W. B. Saunders, 1954), 393–394, for the influence of women's organizations on the nursing profession; O'Neil, *Everyone Was Brave,* 77–106. For dates of some of the women's professional and social reform organizations that formed in the late nineteenth century up until 1920, see Appendix B.

14. Alumnae Association of Bellevue School of Nursing, *The Alumnae Association of the Bellevue School of Nursing* (New York: The Alumnae Association of the Bellevue School of Nursing, 1989), 30; Dock and Stewart, *A Short History of Nursing,* 163, includes the founding dates of alumnae associations; Jamieson and Sewall, *Trends in Nursing History,* 394; Agnes G. Deans and Anne L. Austin, *The History of the Farrand Training School for Nurses* (Detroit: Alumnae Association of the Ferrand Training School for Nurses, 1936), for the history of the Farrand Training School for Nurses; Valerie Hart-Smith, "Lystra Gretter," in *American Nursing: A Biographical Dictionary,* eds. Vern Bullough, Olga Maranjian Church, and Alice P. Stein (New York: Garland Publishing, 1988), 156–58; and a brief history published by the alumnae of the *Harper Hospital School of Nursing 1883–1983* (sent by the alumnae association).

15. Editorial Comment, "The Chicago Conventions," *AJN,* 12 no. 10 (July 1912): 770. The American Federation of Nurses disbanded in 1912 and the American Nurses' Association represented American nursing interests.

16. See appendix I for a listing of those nurse training schools that had opened by 1893.

17. Stella Goostray, "Linda Richards," in James, James, and Boyer, *Notable American Women,* 148–150; Linda Richards, *Reminiscences,* (Boston: Whitcomb and Barrows, 1911. Reprint. Philadelphia: J.B. Lippincott, 1949); Vern L. Bullough, "Linda Ann Judson Richards," in Bullough, Church, and Stein, *American Nursing,* 270–272.

18. Lavinia Dock, "Our Debt to the Woman Movement," *The I.C.N.,* 4 no. 3 (July 1929): 197.

19. Nancy L. Noel, "Isabel Adams Hampton Robb," in Bullough, Church, and Stein, *American Nursing,* 274–6; Isabel Hampton Robb, "The Past, Present, and Future of Nursing in the United States of America," *AJN,* 11 no. 1 (October 1910): 24–6, for the Robb's story of the two boys playing ball; and Mary Jane Rodabaugh, "Isabel Adams Hampton Robb," James, James, and Boyer, *Notable American Women,* 171–2.

20. Janet Wilson James, Biographical Introduction, in *A Lavinia Dock Reader,* ed. Janet Wilson James (New York: Garland Publishing Company, 1985), vii–xix; Sandra Lewenson, "American Nurses: Forging Social Reform in America, Lavinia Dock" (paper delivered at the National Student Nurses' Association 39th Annual Convention, San Antonio, TX, 1991), 1–15; Bullough, Church, and Stein, *American Nursing,* 91–94.

21. Dock and Stewart, *A Short History of Nursing,* 173–6; M. Patricia Donahue, "Mary Adelaide Nutting," in Bullough, Church, and Stein, *American Nursing,* 244–47; Virginia M. Dunbar, "Mary Adelaide Nutting," *Notable American Women,* 642–44.

22. Alumnae Association of Bellevue School of Nursing, *The Alumnae Association of the Bellevue School of Nursing,* 25; Theresa Dombrowski, "Annie Damer," in Bullough, Church, and Stein, *American Nursing,* 74–76.

23. M. Patricia Donahue, "M. Sophia French Palmer," in Bullough, Church, and Stein, *American Nursing,* 252–54; Teresa Christy, "Portrait of a Leader: Sophia F. Palmer," *Nursing Outlook,* 23 (December 1975): 746; Victor Robinson, *White Caps: The Story of Nursing* (Philadelphia: J.B. Lippincott, 1946), 343–44.

24. Althea T. Davis, "Martha Minerva Franklin," in Bullough, Church, and Stein, *American Nursing,* 120–123.

25. Althea Davis, "Adah Belle Samuels Thoms," Bullough, Church, and Stein, *American Nursing,* 313–316.

26. Robert H. Bremner, "Lillian Wald," James, James, and Boyer, *Notable American Women,* 3:526–529; Gerhard Falk, "Lillian Wald," in Bullough, Church, and Stein, *American Nursing,* 331–334; Lillian Wald, *The House on Henry Street,* (New York: Henry Holt and Company, 1915); Lillian Wald, *Windows on Henry Street,* (Boston: Little, Brown, and Company, 1934); New York Hospital Training School for Nurses application blank dated May 11, 1889, for Lillian Wald, Medical Archives, New York Hospital-Cornell Medical Center, Lillian Wald Folder, New York (hereafter called the NYH-CMC); New York Hospital Training School for Nurses application blank dated June 21, 1889, for Mary Brewster, NYH-CMC, New York Hospital Training School Records; and November 13, 1901, minutes of the Alumnae Association of New York Hospital Training School of Nursing, NYH-CMC, p. 200. Little is known of Mary Brewster. However, her married name was Booth, she continued to be active at the Henry Street Settlement House, and she died at a young age after a long illness requiring hospitalization at New York Hospital.

27. See Kenneth S. Mernitz, "Ella Phillips Crandall," in Bullough, Church, and Stein, *American Nursing,* 68–70.

28. Vern Bullough, "Mary Sewall Gardner," in Bullough, Church, and Stein, *American Nursing,* 130–132.

29. Darche, "Employments for Women," *The Delineator,* 668.

30. Darche, ibid.

31. Adelaide Nutting, "The Training of Visiting Nurses," in *A Sound Economic Basis for Schools of Nursing,* 112.

32. North, "A New Profession for Women," 43–46, for a general description of work of the "district nurse" presented in a popular periodical.

33. For references pertaining to the formation of each of the four nursing organizations, see the descriptions of the organizations which appear in the next section of this chapter.

34. For a discussion on women's cooperation in social reform, see Susan Armeny, "Organized Nurses, Women Philanthropists, and the Intellectual Basis for Cooperation Among Women, 1898–1920," in Ellen Condliffe Lagemann, ed., *Nursing History: New Perspectives, New Possibilities* (New York: Teachers College Press, 1983), 13–45; O'Neill, *Everyone Was Brave,* 77–106; for description of reform activism and public health nursing, see Report of the Joint Committee Appointed for Consideration of the Standardization of Visiting Nurses, *AJN,* 12 no. 11 (August 1912): 894–897; for discussion of the reform efforts of women between the 1890s and early 1900s, see Glenda Riley, *Inventing the American Woman: A Perspective on Women's History* (Arlington Heights, Illinois: Harlan Davidson, 1986, 1987), 153–155.

35. The concept of nursing as a window of opportunity for women was presented by Vern Bullough in his presentation on social history at the Fourth Invitational History Conference held at the Nursing Museum, Philadelphia Hospital, Philadelphia, April 1991.

36. Vern Bullough and Bonnie Bullough, *The Emergence of Modern Nursing,* vol. 2 (London: Macmillan Company, 1969), 149, Bullough and Bullough consider the Superintendents' Society to be "the first professional group to be organized and controlled by women in the United States."

37. Evelyn Benson, "Nursing and the World's Columbian Exposition," *Nursing Outlook* 34 no. 2 (March/April, 1986): 88–90; Evelyn Benson, "Nineteenth Century Women, The Neophyte Nursing Profession, and the World's Columbian Exposition of 1893," in Bullough, Bullough, and Stanton, *Florence Nightingale and Her Era,* 108–22; Dock and Stewart, *A*

Short History of Nursing, 241–283; Isabel A. Hampton and others, *Nursing of the Sick 1893* (New York: McGraw-Hill, 1949), xv–xix; Johns S. Billings and Henry M. Hurd, eds., Part III, "Nursing of the Sick," from *Hospitals, Dispensaries and Nursing: Papers and Discussions in the International Congress of Charities, Correction, and Philanthropy, Section III, Chicago, June 12–17th, 1893* (Baltimore: Johns Hopkins Press, 1894). Hampton's book in 1949 was a reissue of Billings and Hurd 1893 edition and was sponsored by the National League for Nursing Education.

38. *The World's Fair, Being a Pictorial History of the Columbian Exposition,* (Syracuse, NY: H.C. Leavenworth and Co., 1893), 4.

39. Ibid., 167, Lois Howe of Boston won second place and Laura Hayes of Chicago won third place for their architectural plans for the Woman's Pavilion; *The World's Fair,* ibid. 210, Bertha Honore Palmer is referred to as Mrs. Potter Palmer in the picture which appears in the front of the book on the exposition; Isabel Ross, "Bertha Honore Palmer," in James, James, and Boyer, *Notable American Women,* III: 10–11; see Frances Willard, "Woman's Department of the World's Fair," in *The World's Fair,* 451–452.

40. A Character Sketch by an Intimate, "Foreign Delegates and Organizations," Ethel Gordon Fenwick, 865, Fenwick was the president of the British nursing section at the Chicago World's Fair; Minnie Goodnow, *Outlines of Nursing History,* 4th ed. (Philadelphia: W.B. Saunders, 1929), 108, 113–15; Elizabeth M. Jamieson and Mary F. Sewall, *Trends in Nursing History: Their Relationships to World Events,* 4th ed. (Philadelphia: W.B. Saunders, 1954), 372, for general histories of nursing that include a brief description of Ethel Gordon Fenwick; Frances Willard, "Woman's Department of the World's Fair," in *The World's Fair,* 468, for description of the British exhibit presented by the London School for Trained Nurses.

41. "Introduction," *First and Second Annual Convention of the American Society of Superintendents of Training Schools* (Harrisburg, PA: Harrisburg Publishing Company, 1897), 3, congresses were described as "international gatherings"; Celia Davies, "Professionalizing Strategies as Time- and Culture-Bound: American and British Nursing, Circa 1893," in Ellen Condliffe Lagemann, ed., *Nursing History: New Perspectives, New Possibilities* (New York: Teachers College Press, 1983), 47–63, for a discussion of the professionalizing strategies of the Superintendents' Society; Jamieson and Sewall, *Trends in Nursing History,* 395–96.

42. Isabel A. Hampton and others, *Nursing of the Sick 1893* (New York: McGraw-Hill, 1949) [sponsored by the NLNE]. This book is a reissue

of Johns S. Billings and Henry M. Hurd, eds., Part III, "Nursing of the Sick," from *Hospitals, Dispensaries and Nursing: Papers and Discussions in the International Congress of Charities, Correction, and Philanthropy, Section III, Chicago, June 12–17th, 1893* (Baltimore: Johns Hopkins Press, 1894); Benson, "Nursing and the World's Columbian Exposition," 89; Benson, "Nineteenth Century Women, The Neophyte Nursing Profession," 117–118.

43. Isabel Stewart, "Introduction," *Nursing of the Sick 1893,* xv.

44. Hampton, *Nursing of the Sick 1893.*

45. Louise Darche, "Proper Organization of Training Schools in America" in Hampton, *Nursing of the Sick 1893,* 93; for historical background of the Superintendents' Society, see Helen Munson, *The Story of the National League for Nursing Education,* 13.

46. Isabel A. Hampton, "Introduction," in First and Second Annual Conventions of the American Society of Superintendents of Training Schools for Nurses, (Harrisburg, PA: 1897), 4; Reverby, *Annual Convention 1893–1899,* 4; Birnbach and Lewenson, *First Words,* xxvi. A list of those in attendance at the first meeting includes:

> Miss Alston, Mt. Sinai Training School, New York, NY
> Miss Betts, Homeopathic Hospital, Brooklyn, NY
> Miss Bannister, Wisconsin Training School, Milwaukee, WI
> Miss Darche, NYC Training School, Blackwell's Island, NY
> Miss Dock, late of Johns Hopkins Hospital, Baltimore, MD
> Miss Davis, University Hospital, Philadelphia, PA
> Miss Greenwood, Jewish Hospital, Cincinnati, OH
> Miss Hampton, Johns Hopkins Hospital, Baltimore, MD
> Miss Lett, St. Luke's Hospital, Chicago, IL
> Miss McKechnie, City Hospital, Louisville, KY
> Miss Nourse, Michael Reese Hospital, Chicago, IL
> Miss Palmer, Garfield Memorial Hospital, Washington, DC
> Miss Sutliffe, New York Hospital, NY
> Miss Somerville, General Hospital, Lawrence, MA
> Miss Wallace, Children's Hospital, San Francisco, CA

47. Nettie Birnbach, "Mary E.P. Davis," In Bullough, Sentz, and Stein, *American Nursing,* 2: 80.

48. Hampton, "Introduction," *Annual Conventions,* p. 4; Birnbach and Lewenson, *First Words,* xxvi; for general history of the Superintendents' Society, see Helen W. Munson, *The Story of the National League for Nursing Education* (Philadelphia: W.B. Saunders, 1934), 13–16.

49. Anna L. Alston, First Convention, *Annual Conventions,* 7.

50. *First and Second Annual Conventions of the ASSTSN* (Harrisburg, PA: Harrisburg, 1897) 7, ANHNC: Anna L. Alston, *Annual Conventions,* 7; Seymer, *A General History of Nursing,* 273–28, for description of the professional nursing journals available in the late 1880s; see Appendix D for a copy of a letter to the superintendents from Anna L. Alston and Louise Darche, 1893, NLN-MS. C 274, History of Medicine Division, National Library of Medicine.

51. "Constitution, Article V," First Convention, *Annual Conventions,* 10.

52. First Convention, ibid.

53. Minutes of the First Annual Convention in *First and Second Annual Conventions,* ANHNC, first convention, and in Reverby, *Annual Conventions,* 10–5. The category of honorary members included those who were so designated by the members of the society; Dolan, *Goodnow's History of Nursing,* 282; Minnie Goodnow, *Outlines of Nursing History,* 4th ed. (Philadelphia: W.B. Saunders, 1929), 454–55, for general history of the Superintendents' Society.

54. Minutes of the First Annual Convention in *First and Second Annual Conventions,* ANHNC, 16; Reverby, *Annual Conventions,* 16.

55. Appendix E "Officers for Next Annual Meeting Appointed or Elected January 11th, 1894," Unpublished minutes of the first convention of the ASSTSN, HMD-NLM, Bethesda, MD, NLN-MS. C 274, Box 2, exhibit 3a; Ida Sutliffe is Irene Sutliffe's younger sister who became superintendent at the Long Island College Hospital School in Brooklyn, NY.

56. Isabel McIssac, Minutes of the First Annual Convention in *First and Second Annual Conventions,* ANHNC, 17; and in Reverby, First Annual, *Annual Conventions,* 17.

57. McIsaac, ibid.

58. Linda Richards, Opening address, Minutes of the First Annual Convention in *First and Second Conventions,* ANHNC, 20; Reverby, First Annual, *Annual Conventions,* 20.

59. Richards, ibid., 22.

60. "A paper was read by Miss Palmer, late superintendent of the Garfield Memorial Hospital" during the third session held on Thursday, February 14, 1895, Unpublished minutes of the Second Annual Convention, NLN-MS. C 274, Box 2, exhibit 3a, p. 43, History of Medicine Division, National Library of Medicine, Bethesda, MD.; Sophia Palmer, "Training School Alumnae Associations," *First and Second Annual Conventions of the American Society of Training Schools for Nurses,* ANHNC, 52–3; and in Reverby, First and Second, *Annual Conventions,* 52–3.

61. Palmer, ibid., 55.

62. Palmer, ibid., 56.

63. See Mary Agnes Snively, "A Uniform Curriculum for Training Schools," *First and Second Annual Convention,* ANHNC, 25; and Reverby, Second Annual, *Annual Conventions,* 25; Although Snively does not mention this, she used an argument similar to one levied against the advancement of women's education earlier in the nineteenth century.

64. Snively, "A Uniform Curriculum," p. 25.

65. Ibid., 27–30, for further discussion of a proposed uniform curriculum.

66. Lavinia L. Dock, "Directories for Nurses," *First and Second Annual Conventions of the ASSTSN,* ANHNC, 57; Reverby, *Annual Conventions,* 57.

67. Dock, "Directories for Nurses," p. 58.

68. Diana Kimber, "Trained Nursing for People of Moderate Incomes," *Fourth Annual Convention of the ASSTSN,* (Harrisburg, PA: Harrisburg Publishing Co., 1897), 25; Reverby, *Annual Conventions,* 25; Kimber explained that a private duty nurse should be able to charge seemingly high fees because trained private duty nurses work "not five hours a day, as teachers do, nor six to eight hours a day, as stenographers and typewriters do, but sixteen, eighteen, twenty and sometimes twenty-four hours a day. Her pay at $21 a week, or $3 a day, is 20 cents an hour for a minimum of fifteen hours, or 15 cents an hour for a maximum of twenty hours' work."

69. Dock, "Directories for Nurses," 57–60; Bullough and Bullough, *The Emergence of Modern Nursing,* 205–206. The 1910 US census reported seven percent of all graduate and student nurses were men. However, throughout the twentieth century a decline in the percentage of males who enter nursing has been observed and is discussed. Dolan, *Goodnow's History of Nursing,* 263, for reference to the low economic value placed on nursing in the hospital. Dolan described how salaries paid to nurses in executive hospital positions indicated their worth to the institution: in 1883 hospitals paid stewards $900 a year, house doctors $1,800, and superintendent of nurses $480.

70. Isabel Hampton Robb, "The Three Years' Course of Training in Connection with the Eight Hour System," *First and Second Annual Conventions of the American Society of Training Schools for Nurses,* ANHNC, 36; Reverby, *Annual Conventions,* 36. Isabel Hampton is hereafter referred to as Isabel Hampton Robb or Mrs. Hunter Robb following her marriage to Dr. Hunter Robb in June 1894.

71. See Linda Richards, "The Superintendent of the Training School," *Fifth Annual Convention of the ASSTSN,* (Harrisburg, PA: Harrisburg Publishing Co., 1898), 51–52; Reverby, *Annual Conventions,* 51–53.

72. Richards, "The Superintendent of the Training School," 53–54.

73. Isabel Hampton Robb, "'Suggestions On Qualifications for Future Membership' in the Society of American Superintendents," *Fifth Annual Convention of the ASSTSN,* (Harrisburg, PA: Harrisburg Publishing Co., 1898), 66–69; Reverby, *Annual Conventions,* 66–69.

74. Adelaide Nutting, *Sixth Annual Convention of the American Society of Superintendents of Training Schools for Nurses* (Harrisburg, PA: Harrisburg Publishing Co., 1900), 64; Reverby, *Annual Conventions,* 64.

75. Nutting, "Sixth Annual Convention," 64.

76. Isabel Hampton Robb, "Educational, Hospital Economics," *AJN,* 1 no. 1 (October 1900): 29–36, presents the requirements, purpose, and syllabus of the lectures for the special course in hospital economics.

77. Bullough and Bullough, *The Emergence of Modern Nursing,* 153–154; Dock and Stewart, *Short History of Nursing,* 175–176; Stewart, *The Education of Nurses,* 145–146, 277; Deborah MacLurg Jenson, *A History of Nursing,* (St. Louis: Mosby, 1943), 183–184; Adelaide Nutting, "Twenty Years of Nursing in Teachers College," *A Sound Economic Basis For Schools of Nursing,* 254–260; Isabel Hampton Robb [Education Committee], *Sixth Annual Convention of the American Society of Superintendents of Training Schools for Nurses,* 57–62; Reverby, *Annual Conventions,* 57–62; "Twenty-Five Years of Nursing Education in Teachers College 1899–1925," *Teachers College Bulletin,* 17th Series, no. 3 (February 1926), iii–58, for history of Teachers College; Robert J. Fridlington, "Helen Hartley Jenkins," James, James, and Boyer, *Notable American Women,* 273–274, for biographical information on Hartley.

78. Burgess, *Nurses, Patients, and Pocketbooks,* 35, for monograph of data collected on the number of nursing schools and trained nurses compared to medical schools and physicians.

79. Genevieve Cooke, Response to Address of Welcome and President's Address, Proceedings of the Seventeenth Annual Convention of the American Nurses' Association, *AJN,* 14 no. 10 (July 1914): 794–798; M.E.P. Davis, "Organization, or Why Belong?," *AJN,* 12, no. 6 (March 1912): 474–477; Isabel Hampton, during a discussion of alumnae associations found in the *First and Second Annual Conventions of the American Society of Training Schools for Nurses* (Harrisburg, PA: Harrisburg Publishing Co., 1897), p. 17, *ANHNC,* New York, for the history of the Associated Alumnae presented in addresses at the meetings of the Superintendents' Society and the Associated Alumnae.

80. Constitution, *Proceedings of Convention of Training School Alumnae Delegates and Representatives from the American Society of Superintendents of*

Training Schools for Nurses held at Manhattan Beach Hotel, September 2–4, 1896 (Harrisburg, PA: Harrisburg Publishing Co., 1896), 20–1. NLN-MS. C 274, HMD, NLM, Bethesda, MD. According to the constitution of the fledgling association in 1896, active membership consisted of "delegates duly elected to represent the Alumnae Associations belonging to this Association."

81. Dock, "A National Association for Nurses and its Legal Organization," *Third Annual Convention of The American Society of Superintendents of Training Schools for Nurses,* 42–60, ANHNC, New York; Reverby, *Annual Conventions,* 42–60.

82. Dock, "A National Association for Nurses," 42–60.

83. Ibid., Dock considered New York State most likely to grant a charter for the national association because the state had the largest number of training schools.

84. Ibid., 47.

85. Ibid., 59.

86. See comment by Miss Walter (Miss Walker as per errata note in Index) in the discussion following Dock's paper, "A National Association for Nurses and its Legal Organization," see *Third Annual Convention of ASSTSN,* 64; Reverby, *Annual! Conventions,* 64.

87. Discussion following Dock's paper, "A National Association for Nurses and its Legal Organization," see *Third Annual Convention of ASSTSN,* 63–64; Reverby, *Annual Conventions,* 63–64.

88. Committee on the National Association report, *Fourth Annual Convention of the ASSTSN* (Harrisburg, PA: Harrisburg Publishing Co., 1897), 12; Reverby, *Annual Conventions,* 12; for names of the members selected to form the constitutional committee, see *Proceedings of Convention Training School Alumnae Delegates and Representatives from the ASSTSN* (Harrisburg, PA: Harrisburg Publishing Co., 1896), NLN-MS. C 274, HMD, NLM, Box 6, p. 23.

89. M.E.P. Davis, "Organization, or Why Belong?," *AJN,* 12 no. 6 (1912): 474–477; Proceedings of Convention Training School Alumnae Delegates and Representatives from the ASSTSN (Harrisburg, PA: Harrisburg Publishing Co., 1896), NLN-MS. C 274, HMD, NLM, Box 6, p. 12. The following delegates and superintendents from alumnae associations were present at the roll call taken at the first session on Wednesday, September 2nd, 1897, at 2:30 p.m., Phoebe Brown, delegate, Illinois Training School; Ella Clapp, delegate, New Haven Training School; J.R. Hawley, delegate, Philadelphia Training School; Anna Maxwell, Superintendent Presbyterian Training School; Margaret A.

Mullen, delegate, Garfield Training School; H. Morand, delegate, University of Pennsylvania Training School; Sophia Palmer, Superintendent Rochester Hospital; Bessie Pierson, delegate, Orange Memorial Training School; Miss Ross, delegate, Johns Hopkins Training School; M.W. Stevenson, delegate, Massachusetts General Training School; Mary E. Smith, delegate, Farrand Training School; Lucy Walker, Superintendent Pennsylvania Training School; and Lena Walden, delegate, New York Training School.

90. *Proceedings of Convention Training School Alumnae Delegates and Representatives from the ASSTSN,* 5–9.

91. *Proceedings of Convention,* ibid., 15.

92. Undated and unnamed newspaper clipping one week before the February 10, 11, and 12, 1897, meeting of the Superintendents' Society, "To Meet Here Next Week The American Society of Superintendents of Training Schools for Nurses," NLN-MS. C 274, HMD, NLM, Box 6.

93. For unpublished minutes of the Nurses' Associated Alumnae, see Unpublished minutes of the First Annual Meeting held April 28–29, 1898 in New York, MML-NA, Box 33; see Mary E. P. Davis, "Organization, or Why Belong," *AJN,* 12 no. 6 (March 1912): 474–477; the United States had just declared war with Spain on April 21, 1898.

94. Dolan, *Goodnow's History of Nursing,* 250–252; Goodnow, *Outlines of Nursing History,* 147–154; Kalisch and Kalisch, *The Advance of American Nursing,* 195–223, for discussion of nursing's role in the Spanish-American War.

95. See Susan Armeny, "Organized Nurses, Women Philanthropists, and the Intellectual Bases for Cooperation Among Women, 1898–1920," in Ellen Condliffe Lagemann, ed., *Nursing History, New Perspectives, New Possibilities,* (New York: Teachers College Press, 1893), 13–24, for critical essay concerning the relationship among McGee and the Daughters of the American Revolution, the American Red Cross, and the Associated Alumnae during the Spanish-American War; see Mary R. Dearing, "Anita Newcomb McGee," James, James, and Boyer, *Notable American Women,* 464–66; Cindy Gurney and Dolores J. Haritos, "Anita Newcomb McGee," *American Nursing,* 217–220, for description of McGee's input during the Spanish-American War.

96. "Board of Directors Minutes 1897–1929," unpublished minutes of meeting held on December 28, 1898, at the New York Training School in New York, MML-NA, Convention Proceedings, Box 33, Folder 1, p. 18. The minutes of the December 28, 1898, meeting also reflected the board's discussion of a proposed army training school for

nurses and the pay for each of the suggested positions for nurses serving in the army.

97. The American National Association of the Red Cross (hereafter referred to as the American Red Cross) was officially founded in 1882 and Civil War nurse Clara Barton (1821–1912) was its president. The New York branch of independent workers which formed the Red Cross Relief Committee included wealthy New Yorkers. They organized auxiliary groups to provide relief services throughout the Spanish-American war.

98. Armeny, *Nursing History: New Perspectives,* 20; Goodnow, *Outlines of Nursing History,* 147–154; Kalisch and Kalisch, *The Advance of American Nursing,* 195–223; *see* Sarah Elizabeth Pickett, *The American National Red Cross, Its Origin, Purposes, and Service,* (New York: The Century Co., 1923), 14–16, for the history of the American Red Cross.

99. Armeny, *Nursing History: Nursing Perspective,* 18–23; Joan LeB. Downer, "Anna Caroline Maxwell," in Bullough, Church, and Stein, *American Nursing,* 232–236.

100. Isabel Hampton Robb, "Original Communications, Address of the President," *AJN,* 1 no. 2 (November 1900): 97.

101. Ibid., 99.

102. Ibid.

103. Ibid.

104. Robb, ibid. Robb does not identify by name the group of women that she refers to as commercial. However, using Armeny's theses and the outcomes of this episode in history, Robb may be referring to the Daughters of the American Revolution and Dr. McGee as the commercial women who were untrained in nursing and lacked understanding of the trained nurses.

105. Ibid., 108; the Army Nurses Corps legislation, which ensured a permanent supply of trained nurses in the army during peacetime as well as wartime, was passed in 1901; a similar bill providing a Navy Nurses Corps passed in 1908; *see* Jamieson and Sewall, *Trends in Nursing History,* 403; and Kalisch and Kalisch, *Advance of American Nursing,* 217–220; and undated and unnamed newspaper clipping, "The Nursing World," NLN-MS. C 274, HMD-NLM, Bethesda, MD, Box 6, p. 40, for history regarding the creation of the Army Nurses Corps.

106. International Council of Women, *Women In A Changing World: The Dynamic Story of the International Council of Women Since 1888* (London: Routledge and Kegan Paul, 1966), 3–39, for the history of International

Council of Women between 1888 and 1914; Clifton J. Phillips, "May Eliza Wright Sewall," in James, James, and Boyer, *Notable American Women,* 268–269; Linda E. Sabin, "Clara (Clarissa Harlowe) Barton," Bullough, Church, and Stein, *American Nursing,* 16–19; Merle Curti, "Barton, Clara," James, James, and Boyer, *Notable American Women,* 103–8); The American Red Cross, *Clara Barton and Dansville* (Dansville, NY: privately published, 1966).

107. *International Council of Women Handbook,* 2nd ed. (1899). *Handbook of the International Congress-Program of Quinquennial Meetings of the International Council of Women,* 2nd ed. (1899) p. 57, located in envelope marked p. 13, NLN-MS. C 274, HMD-NLM, Box 6, Bethesda; see Cott, *The Grounding of Modern Feminism,* 255; Irwin, *Angels and Amazons,* Appendix 443–499, for description of the ICW and the NCW; see D.C. Bridges, *A History of the International Council of Nurses, 1899–1964,* (Philadelphia: Lippincott, 1967), for general description of the International Council of Nurses and for the relationship between American nursing organizations and the woman's movement through their affiliation with the ICN.

108. Lavinia Dock, "The International Council of Nurses," *AJN,* 1 no. 2 (November 1900): 114; the Matron's Council had formed a provisional committee to form the International Council of Nurses. Dock includes the constitution written by the provisional committee and adopted in July 1900 in London; Editorial, "1899–July-1929," *The ICN,* 9 no. 3 (July 1929): 14–151. According to the editorial, the International Council of Nurses was considered the oldest of the International organizations to be established by a professional group of workers. Other international professional councils to form included the International Dental Federation in 1900, the International Society of Surgeons in 1902, the International Pharmaceutical Federation in 1912, the International Association in Midwives in 1925, and the International Professional Medical Association in 1926.

109. Margaret Breay and Ethel Gordon Fenwick, *History of the International Council of Nurses, 1899–1925* (Geneva: The ICN, 1931), 59.

110. Breay and Fenwick, ibid., 59. Dock, *Short History of Nursing,* 344–346, for description of the International Council of Nurses; *Fourth Annual Convention of the American Society of Superintendents of Training Schools for Nurses,* (Harrisburg, PA: Harrisburg Publishing Co., 1897), 13 and 37; Reverby, *Annual Conventions,* 13 and 37, for letter sent to the Superintendents' Society and the selection of delegates Draper and Smith; see *Fifth Annual Convention of the American Society of Superintendents of Training Schools for Nurses,* (Harrisburg, PA: Harrisburg Publishing Co.,

1898), 11; Reverby, *Annual Conventions,* 11, for Snively's concern for cost of sending delegates.

111. Letter addressed to Miss F. Isaac from the President of the National Council of Women (unsigned) dated December 17, 1898, unpublished letter, NLN-MS. C 274, HMD-NLM, Box 6, p. 47. The president of the Superintendents' Society was Isabel McIsaac; however, the letter was addressed to Miss F. Isaac.

112. Ibid.

113. *Seventh Annual Convention of The American Society of Superintendents of Training Schools for Nurses,* (Harrisburg, PA: Harrisburg Publishing Co., 1900), 29–33, for a discussion in the minutes concerning membership in the NCW.

114. Letter to Miss L.L. Dock from May Wright Sewall, dated February 23, 1900 [summary], in the *Seventh Annual Convention of the American Society of Superintendents of Training Schools for Nurses* (Harrisburg, PA: Harrisburg Publishing Co., 1900), 30–32.

115. Fannie Humphries Gafney and Kate Waller Barrett, *Seventh Annual Convention of the Superintendents' Society,* 109.

116. See Extracts from Draft Constitution of International Council of Nurses, *Seventh Annual Convention of the Superintendents' Society,* 110.

117. See Extracts from Draft Constitution of International Council of Nurses, Memorandum, *Seventh Annual Convention of the Superintendents' Society,* 111.

118. Bedford Fenwick, *Seventh Annual Convention of the Superintendents' Society,* 111.

119. See Second Annual Convention of the Associated Alumnae, May 2, 1899, afternoon session, Unpublished proceedings, "Board of Directors Minutes 1897–1929," MML-NA, N87; Convention proceedings, Box 33, Folder 1; however, the unpublished minutes show none of the discussions or decisions on the subject.

120. Robb, "Original Communications: Address of the President," 103.

121. For listing of the quinquennial ICW meetings and the names of the countries and presidents of the host National Council of Women for these meetings, see International Council of Women, *Women in a Changing World: The Dynamic Story of the International Council of Women Since 1888,* (London: Routledge, & Kegan Paul, 1966), 349; The ICN held its meetings every five years. Hence the quinquennial meetings following the first foundation meeting in Washington, D.C. in 1888:

1. Chicago, Illinois
2. London, England
3. Berlin, Germany
4. Toronto, Canada
5. Rome, Italy
6. Christiania (Oslo, Norway)

122. Comment by Lavinia Dock in the "Report of the Third Annual Convention of the Associated Alumnae of Trained Nurses," *AJN,* 1 no. 1 (1900): 76.

123. Ibid., 76; see unnamed and undated newspaper clipping, "The Nursing World," NLN-MS. C 274, HMD-NLM, Bethesda, MD, Box 6, p. 40.

124. See, "Report of the Third Annual Convention of the Associated Alumnae of Trained Nurses" *AJN,* 1 no. 1 (1900): 77. The committee selected to study affiliation between the Superintendents' Society and the Associated Alumnae included Lavinia Dock from Bellevue; Miss Graham from New York Post-Graduate; Miss Brobson from the University of Pennsylvania; Miss Thornton from the Farrand Training School, and Jessie Breeze from Illinois selected as chair.

125. Third Annual Convention of the NAA May 3–5, 1900, Unpublished proceedings, "Board of Directors Minutes 1897–1929," MML, NA, N 87, Convention proceedings, Box 33, Folder 1, pp. 41–59; Letter dated October 4, 1900 addressed "Dear Madam" from Lavinia Dock, NLN-MS. C 274, HMD-NLM, Bethesda, MD, Box 6, p. 44, for announcement that affiliation between the Superintendents' Society and the Associated Alumnae for the purpose of entering the National Council of Women was approved.

126. Unpublished minutes of Superintendents' Society dated Detroit, June 1902, and signed L.L. Dock, secretary, NLN-MS. C 274, HMD-NLM, Box 2, exhibit 3a, p. 99; Lystra Gretter, *Ninth Annual Convention of the ASSTSN* (Harrisburg, PA: Harrisburg Publishing Co., 1902), 6–7.

127. Lena Dufton ed., *History of Nursing at New York Post-Graduate Medical School and Hospital* (New York: The Alumnae Association, 1944), 71–2; Unpublished minutes of the Fourth Annual Convention of the Nurses' Associated Alumnae, 1901 September 16th and 17th, MML, Box 33, p. 70. Mary Thornton along with Miss Healy was selected by Isabel Hamptom Robb to represent the Nurses' Associated Alumnae at the American Federation of Nurses.

128. See Lavinia Dock, Report from Committee on Affiliation with the National Council of Women at the Eighth Annual Meeting of the

ASSTSN, held on September 16, 1901, p. 96, Unpublished proceedings, NLN-MS. C 274, HMD-NLM, Box 2, Exhibit 3a, p. 96.

129. See Emma J. Keating, Report as delegate to the National Council of Women, *Proceedings of the Eighth Annual Convention of the ASSTSN* (held in 1901) (Harrisburg, PA: Harrisburg Publishing Co., 1902), 17–18.

130. Report of The American Federation of Nurses, *AJN*, 4 no. 8 (May 1904): 619.

131. Ibid., 621.

132. "Busy Day for Nurses," *Washington Post,* May 1905 (date unknown), p. 84, NLN-MS. C 274, HMD-NLM, Box 6; Lucy Ridgely Seymer, *A General History of Nursing* (New York, The Macmillan Co., 1933), 270. American nursing representatives had attended the International Council of Nurses first quinquennial meeting in Berlin, Germany, in 1904, and was one of three countries (the other two were Great Britain and Germany) to have a national organization affiliated. However, Seymer does not mention the American Federation of Nurses.

133. Lavinia Dock, "International Relationships," *Eleventh Annual Report of ASSTSN Including Report of the First Meeting of the American Federation of Nurses* (Baltimore: J.H. Furst Co. 1905), 169–176; Unpublished Minutes of Council Meeting of the Superintendents' Society, April 30, 1905, Unpublished proceedings, NLN-MS. C 274, HMD-NLM, Box 2, Exhibit 3b, 187–8. In preparation for the Superintendents' Society convention, a joint meeting with the Associated Alumnae constituting the first meeting of the American Federation of Nurses was planned for the 1905 annual convention. There they planned to discuss "affiliation with the International Council of Nurses" and "also that of withdrawing from the National Council of Women."

134. Ibid., 176.

135. Ibid.

136. Editorial Comment, "The Chicago Conventions," *AJN*, 12 no. 10 (July 1912): 770; Unpublished Minutes of Council Meeting of the Superintendents' Society, January 12, 1912, held in Nutting's office, Unpublished proceedings, NLN-MS. C 274, HMD-NLM, Box 2, Exhibit 3b, 254. The American Federation of Nurses disbanded in 1912 and the American Nurses' Association represented American nursing interests to the international community.

137. Dock and Stewart, *A Short History of Nursing,* 170. Dock and Stewart described the *AJN* as a "professional organ," published and edited by nurses for professional reasons instead of financial or literary reasons; Kalisch and Kalisch, *Advance of American Nursing,* 142–143. Prior to

1900 four nursing periodicals in America existed: *The Nightingale,* published between 1886–1891; *The Trained Nurse and Hospital Review,* first published in August 1888 and lasting more than seventy years; *The Nursing Record,* and *The Nursing World,* both published during the late 1890s.

138. Editorial Comment, "An Anniversary," *AJN,* 10 no. 12 (September 1910). 928.

139. Genevieve Cooke, "Response to Address of Welcome and President's Address, Proceedings of the Seventeenth Annual Convention of the ANA," *AJN,* 14 no. 10 (1914): 794–798; Lavinia Dock, *A History of Nursing from the Earliest Times to the Present Day with Special Reference to the Work of the Past Thirty Years,* vol. 3 (New York: G.P. Putnam's Sons, 1912); Editorial Comment, *AJN,* 10 no. 12 (September 1910):928–929.

140. Clara Noyes, Editorial Comment, "The Fifteenth Birthday of the Journal," *AJN,* 16 no. 1 (October, 1915): 1–9.

141. Editorial Comment, "The Chicago Conventions," 771.

142. See "The Editor," *AJN,* 1 no. 1 (October, 1900): 64.

143. Dock, *A History of Nursing,* 3:200.

144. "The Editor," 65.

145. Editorial Comment, "An Anniversary," 929.

146. Darlene Clark Hine, "Origins of the Black Hospital and Nurse Training School Movement," and "Racism, Status, and the Professionalization of Black Nursing," in *Black Women In White: Racial Conflict and Cooperation in the Nursing Profession, 1890–1950,* (Bloomington: Indiana University Press, 1989), 1–25, 89–107, for an in-depth discussion illustrating the struggles African-American women faced as women and as nurses in America during the modern nursing movement; Darlene Clark Hine, "The Ethel Johns Report: Black Women in the Nursing Profession, 1925," and "From Hospital to College: Black Nurse Leaders and the Rise of Collegiate Nursing Schools," in *Black Women in United States History,* vol. 2 of the *Black Women in American History: The Twentieth Century,* ed. Darlene Clark Hine (Brooklyn, NY: Carlson Publishing, 1990), 212–228 and 222–337 respectively; Ethel Johns, "A Study of the Present Status of the Negro Woman in Nursing," (1925), AC, RG 1.1, Series 200, Box 122, Folder 1507, pp. 1–43, Exhibits A-P, Appendix I and II; Mabel Staupers, "The Negro Nurse in America," *Opportunity: Journal of Negro Life,* 15 (November 1937), 339–341, 349 and reprinted in Darlene Clark Hine, *Black Women in the Nursing Profession: A Documentary History,* (New York: Garland Publishing Co., 1985), 125–27.

147. Hine, "Racism, Status, and the Professionalization of Black Nurses," in *Black Women in White,* 95; Ethel Johns, "A Study of the Present Status of the Negro Woman in Nursing," (1925), Letter to Ethel Johns from Petra Pinn, president of the National Association of Colored Graduate Nurses dated November 15, [1925], RAC, RC, RG 1.1, Series 200, Box 122, Folder 1507, Appendix I.

148. Adah Thoms, *Pathfinders: A History of the Progress of the Colored Graduate Nurses,* (New York: Kay Printing House, 1929); Hine, "Origins of the Black Hospital and Nurse Training School Movement," *Black Women in White,* 1–25.

149. August 25, 1908, unpublished proceedings of the NACGN, the New York Public Library, Schomburg Center for Research in Black Culture, Rare Books, Manuscripts and Archives Section, National Association of Colored Graduate Nurses Records (1908–1951), Box 1, Volume 1, New York (hereafter cited as NACGNR, Schomburg). Notes from the unpublished minutes of the NACGN mention interesting papers on community health but do not include titles or the full address.

150. "Official Reports, New York, N.Y.," *AJN,* 9 no. 2 (November 1908): 144–145.

151. "Official Reports," ibid.; New York Hospital Training School for Nurses application blank dated May 15, 1888, for Jane Hitchcock, Medical Archives, New York Hospital Cornell Medical Center, New York Hospital Training School Records, New York, for Hitchcock's birthdate; Hines, "Racism, Status, and the Professionalization of Black Nursing," *Black Women in White,* 92; Johns, "A Study of the Present Status of the Negro Woman in Nursing," RAC, RC, RG 1.1, Series 200, Box 122, Folder 1508, Appendix I. Lillian Wald was instrumental in the organization of the National Organization of Public Health Nursing which formed four years later in 1912. In the public health organization, women of color were accepted as members because membership into the organization did not rely on association membership.

152. "Official Reports," 144.

153. Thoms, *Pathfinders,* 237.

154. Unpublished proceedings of the NACGN, August 25, 1908, NACGNR, Schomburg, Box 1, Volume 1, p. 13.

155. *For the Health of A Race,* Manuscript Collections Center For the Study of History of Nursing, Mercy-Douglas Hospital MC 78, Series II Mercy Hospital, 1919–1948, University of Pennsylvania, Philadelphia.

156. John A. Kenney, "Some Facts Concerning Negro Nurse Training Schools and Their Graduates," *Journal of the National Medical Association,* 11 (April–June, 1919): 53–68 and reprinted in Hine, *Black Women in the Nursing Profession,* 11. By 1919, Spelman had graduated sixty-three nurses.

157. Staupers, "The Negro Nurse in America," *Opportunity Journal of Negro Life,* 339; "Northern Black Hospitals and Training Schools" and "Training Nurses in Southern Black Hospitals" in Hine, *Black Women in White,* 26–46, 47–62; Hine, *Black Women in White,* 27, the nurse training school at Dixie Hospital and at Hampton Institute affiliated; Manuscript Collections Center for the Study of History of Nursing, The History of Mercy-Douglas Hospital, Mercy-Douglas Hospital Records 1896–1968, MC 78, University of Pennsylvania, Philadelphia. The Frederick Douglass Memorial Hospital Nurse Training School and the Mercy Hospital School of Nursing in Philadelphia merged into the Mercy-Douglas Hospital School of Nursing between 1949 and 1960; Booker T. Washington, "Training Colored Nurses at Tuskagee," *AJN,* 11 no. 3 (December 1910): 167–171.

158. The ten schools and the number of nurses who graduated from each school by 1928 is shown in the following table:

TABLE 2.1

Nurses of Color Who Graduated from Nurse Training by 1928

SCHOOL	LOCATION	GRADUATED BY 1928
LINCOLN HOSPITAL	NEW YORK CITY	496 nurses
FREEDMEN'S HOSPITAL	WASHINGTON, DC	439 nurses
DIXIE-HAMPTON	HAMPTON, VIRGINIA	281 nurses
PROVIDENT HOSPITAL	CHICAGO, ILLINOIS	226 nurses
HUBBARD HOSPITAL	NASHVILLE, TENNESSEE	138 nurses
THE HOSPITAL AND TRAINING SCHOOL OF CHARLESTON	CHARLESTON, SOUTH CAROLINA	127 nurses
MERCY HOSPITAL	PHILADELPHIA, PENNSYLVANIA	136 nurses
ST. AGNES HOSPITAL	RALEIGH, NORTH CAROLINA	172 nurses
FLINT-GOODRICH HOSPITAL	NEW ORLEANS	137 nurses
TUSKEGEE INSTITUTE	TUSKEGEE, ALABAMA	128 nurses

Figures used in this chart were taken from Anna Coles, "The Howard University School of Nursing in Historical Perspective," in Hine, *Black Women in the Nursing Profession,* 29.

159. Minutes of the Rockefeller Foundation dated 21 May 1924, Negro Nursing Education 24107, RAC, RC, RG 1.1, Series 200, Box 121, Folder 1504.

160. Donolda R. Hamlin, "Report on Informal Study of the Educational Facilities for Colored Nurses and Their Use in Hospital, Visiting, and Public Health Nursing" (Chicago, IL: The Hospital Library and Service Bureau, 1924–1925), and reprinted in Hine, *Black Women in the Nursing Profession*, 45–6; Letter dated April 23, 1924, from Donolda Hamlin (letter sent to training schools asking for assistance to the survey), RAC, RC. RG 1.1, Series 200, Box 122, Folder 1505.

161. Ibid., 56.

162. Ibid., 52.

163. Ibid.

164. Ibid.

165. Ibid., 54, for listing of states with schools for black nurses.

166. Hine, *Black Women in White,* 91–2; Birnbach, "The Genesis of the Nurse Registration Movement in the United States, 1893–1903," 21–60.

167. Hine, "Racism, Status, and the Professionalization of Black Nursing," 92–93.

168. Letter from Lucy Hale Topley to the NACGN tenth annual meeting held on August 21, 1917, Unpublished proceedings, NACGNR, Schomburg, Box 1, Volume 2, p. 2.

169. Letter to George E. Vincent (president of the Rockefeller Foundation) from Lucy Hale Topley (president of Spelman College) dated October 7, 1925. Topley agreed to participate in the Ethel Johns Report sponsored by the Rockefeller Foundation. RAC, RC, RG 1.1, Series 200, Box 121, Folder 1505.

170. Johns, "A Study of the Present Status of the Negro Woman in Nursing," RAC, RC, RG 1.1, Series 200, Box 122, Folder 1507. Discriminatory hiring practices of hospitals, private duty, and public health agencies can be observed throughout the Ethel Johns report.

171. Stanley Rayfield, "A Study of Negro Public Health Nursing, Compiled on the Basis of Reports and Statistics Collected by Majory Stimson and Louise Tattershall of the National Organization for Public Health Nursing," in Hine, *Black Women in the Nursing Profession,* 74, and reprinted from the *Public Health Nurse* (October 1930): 525–536; Jessie C. Sleet, "Progressive Movements [in charge of Lucy L. Drown], A Successful Experiment," *AJN,* 1 no. 10 (July 1901): 729–731. Jessie C.

Sleet Scales (1875–1950) published her account of her experimental work as first African-American public health nurse in New York.

172. Rayfield, "A Study of Negro Public Health Nursing," 74; the city is unnamed in the findings. Hine, *Black Women in White*, 8, 10 for description of the Julius Rosenwald Fund established by philanthropist and president of Sears, Roebuck and Company, Julius Rosenwald (1862–1936). During the late nineteenth and early twentieth centuries Rosenwald and other philanthropists such as John D. Rockefeller and Andrew Carnegie donated large sums of money to establish black hospitals and formal nurse training schools for black women. The Rockefeller Foundation, in addition to supporting schools of nursing, sponsored the unpublished Ethel Johns report, "A Study of the Present Status of the Negro Woman in Nursing."

173. Minutes of the Tenth Annual Meeting, 1917, Unpublished proceedings, NACGNR, Schomburg, Box 1, Volume 2, p. 21; Report on the National Registry by Adah Thoms at the eleventh annual meeting of the NACGN on August 20, 1919, found in the Unpublished proceedings, NACGNR, Schomburg, Box 1, Volume 2, p. 33.

174. Minutes of the NACGN executive board meeting held December 3, 1918, Unpublished proceedings, NACGNR, Schomburg, Box 1, Volume 2, p. 51–52; Johns, "A Study of the Present Status of the Negro Woman in Nursing," (1925), RAC, RC, RG 1.1, Series 200, Box 122, Folder 1507, pp. H-8, K-12, for examples of pay inequities between black and white nurses.

175. Pickett, *The American National Red Cross,* 45.

176. Minutes of the Eleventh Annual Meeting, August 20 and 21, 1918, Unpublished proceedings, NACGNR, Schomburg, Box 1, Volume 2, p. 52.

177. Minutes of the Eleventh Annual Meeting, on August 20 and 21, 1918, Unpublished proceedings, NACGNR, Schomburg, Box 1, Volume 2, p. 38. However, the unpublished proceedings do not go into detail as to the arguments for or against African-American nurses serving in World War I or what the NACGN was specifically doing to remedy this situation.

178. Minutes of the Eleventh Annual Meeting, August 20 and 21, 1918, Unpublished proceedings, NACGNR, Schomburg, Box 1, Volume 2, p. 38.

179. Letter sent to NACGN from the eighteen army nurses at the twelfth annual convention of the NACGN convened in Boston, MA, August

19, 1919, Unpublished proceedings, NACGNR, Schomburg, Box 1, Volume 2, p. 58–59.

180. Hines, *Black Women In White,* 94, 104, and Darlene Clark Hines, "The Call That Never Came: Black Women Nurses and World War I, an Historical Note," *Black Women in United States,* 25, reprinted from *Indiana Military History Journal,* 15 (January, 1983), for discussion of the Blue Circle Nurses and the Circle for Negro War Relief.

181. Kalisch and Kalisch, *Advance of American Nursing,* 251–3; Fannie F. Clement, "Town and Country Nursing Service," *AJN,* 15 no. 5 (February 1915): 494–96; "Informal Statement Concerning the Object and Scope of the National Organization for Public Health Nursing and Its Relation to the Red Cross Town and Country Nursing Service," dated November 5, 1915, RAC, RC, RG 1.1, Series 200, Folder 1498, for further reading on the American Red Cross Town and Country Nursing Service; Susan B. DelBene and Vern L. Bullough, "Frances Elliot Davis," in *American Nursing,* 76–78; Joyce Ann Elmore, "Frances Elliot Davis," in Sicherman and Green, *Notable American Women,* 180–82; Hine, *Black Women in White,* 134–36.

182. Ethel Johns, "A Study of the Present Status of the Negro Woman in Nursing," RAC, RC, RG 1.1, Series 200, Box 122, Folder 1507, 29–31 and Exhibit A-18 for the hiring practices of the Henry Street Settlement which was noted as "twenty-five colored nurses as compared with one hundred and fifty white nurses" representing one-sixth of the total staff. Both white and black nurses were equally paid $1,400 per annum. For further background on the public health movement in America, see next section.

183. Kalisch and Kalisch, *Advances in American Nursing,* 558–9, for discussion of health among black Americans; Hine, *Black Women in White,* 188–189; most black nurses worked in private duty or public health positions prior to the 1960s because few jobs were available to them in hospitals; Karen Buhler-Wilkerson, "Caring in Its 'Proper Place': Race and Benevolence in Charleston, SC, 1813–1930," *Nursing Research* 41 (January/February 1992): 13–16, for the discriminatory hiring pattern of the black, public health nurse Anna DeCosta Banks in the Ladies Benevolent Society in Charleston, South Carolina, between 1903 and 1930.

184. Lavinia Dock, "Report of the Thirteenth Annual Convention," *AJN,* 10 no. 11 (August 1910): 902.

185. Ibid.

186. Mabel K. Staupers, "Story of the National Association of Colored Graduate Nurses," in Hine, *Black Women in the Nursing Profession,* 141–44, reprinted from the *AJN,* 51 (April 1951): 222–23; Mabel K. Staupers, *No Time For Prejudice,* (New York: Macmillan Co., 1961).

187. See Adah Thoms, Minutes of the Thirteenth Annual Convention of August 17, 1920 held in Tuskegee, Alabama, Unpublished proceedings, NACGNR, Schomburg, Box 1, Volume 2, p. 84.

188. Ibid., p. 88.

189. Ibid. The minutes did not reflect what Thoms had said or meant by "express[ing] herself freely."

190. Mary E. Carnegie and Estelle M. Osborn, "Integration in Professional Nursing," *Crisis,* 69 (January 1962): 5–9 and in *International Nursing Review,* 9 (August 1962): 47–50, and reprinted in Hine, *Black Women in the Nursing Profession,* 145–148; Staupers, "Story of the National Association of Colored Graduate Nurse," 222–223; Staupers, *No Time for Prejudice.*

191. Hines, "'We Shall Not Be Left Out:' World War II and Integration of Nursing," in *Black Women in White,* 162–186, for the struggle of black nurses for entry into the American military; Staupers, *Story of the National Association of Colored Graduate Nurses,* 142–3; Kenneth S. Mernitz, "Frances Payne Bingham Bolton," in Bullough, Church, and Stein, *American Nursing,* 42–6. Frances Payne Bolton was a philanthropist and benefactor of the NACGN who supported its efforts to break down racial bias in American nursing. Bolton, in 1940, following the death of her husband in 1939, succeeded him and won the congressional seat from Ohio in the U.S. House of Representatives.

192. Carnegie and Osborn, "Integration in Professional Nursing," 146–47; Staupers, *Story of the National Association of Colored Graduate Nurses,* 143–144.

193. Staupers, "Story of the National Association of Colored Graduate Nurses," 144.

194. Staupers, ibid., 144.

195. Charles E. Rosenberg and Carrol Smith-Rosenberg, "Pietism and the Origins of the American Public Health Movement: A Note on John H. Griscom and Robert M. Hartley"; Gert H. Brieger, "Sanitary Reform in New York City: Stephen Smith and the Passage of the Metropolitan Health Bill," in Judith Walzer Leavitt and Ronald Numbers, eds., *Sickness and Health in America: Readings in the History of Medicine and Public Health,* 2nd ed., rev. (Madison, WI: University of Wisconsin Press, 1985), 385–398 and 399–413.

196. The Committee for the Study of Nursing Education, *Nursing and Nursing Education in the United States,* 39–43; Bullough and Bullough, *The Emergence of Modern Nursing,* 156–164; Dacre Craven, *A Guide to District Nurses* (London: Macmillan and Co., 1889), B-23; Nancy Rothman, "Toward Description: Public Health Nursing and Community Health Nursing Are Different," *Nursing and Health Care,* 11 no. 9 (November 1990): 482–483; Buhler-Wilkerson, "Caring in its 'Proper Place': Race and Benevolence in Charleston, SC, 1813–1930," 14, for a description of the Ladies Benevolent Society of Charleston, South Carolina, considered one of the oldest home-based nursing care organizations in America. The term public health nurse was first used by Lillian Wald and included the visiting nurse, the school nurse, and the industrial nurse. The English visiting nurse was called a district nurse.

197. Diane Hamilton, "Research and Reform: Community Nursing and the Framingham Tuberculosis Project, 1914–1923," *Nursing Research,* 41 no. 1 (January/February 1992): –13, describes the innovative use of public health nurses in the Metropolitan Life Insurance Company.

198. Burgess, *Nurses, Patients, and Pocketbooks,* 266, for comments made by public health nurses about the differences between public health nursing and private duty nursing.

199. Ibid., 267.

200. Ibid.

201. Ibid.

202. Ibid., 267. In this same response to Burgess's 1928 study, the public health nurse from California expressed that nursing in that setting permitted her "to keep up with one's clothes, to take an extension course; time to manicure one's nails, [and] to vote and to know why . . . ."

203. Ibid., 266.

204. Stewart, *The Education of Nurses: Historical Foundations and Modern Trends,* 194. The public health movement and the new role of the public health nurse influenced the inclusion of a public health component in nursing education.

205. Nutting, "The Training of Visiting Nurses," *A Sound Economic Basis For Schools of Nursing,* 119.

206. Louise Fitzpatrick, "A History of the National Organization for Public Health Nursing: 1912–1952" Ed.D. diss. Teachers College, Columbia University, 1972, 3–27; Judith Walzer Leavitt, "Politics and Public Health: Smallpox in Milwaukee, 1894–1895," in *Sickness and Health in America,* 372–382; Brieger, "Sanitary Reform in New York City:

Stephen Smith and the Passage of the Metropolitan Health Bill," *Sickness and Health in America,* 399–413; the bacteriological discoveries of scientists such as Ignatz Semmelweis (1818–1865) (aseptic childbirth technique); Louis Pasteur (1822–1895) (smallpox); Joseph Lister (1827–1912); Klebs and Loefter (diphtheria); Welch (gas gangrene); and Koch (tuberculosis) contributed to the public health movement in America in the nineteenth and twentieth century.

207. North, "A New Profession for Women," 43.

208. Nutting, "Nursing and the Public Health," *A Sound Economic Basis For Schools of Nursing,* 148.

209. Wald, *The House on Henry Street,* v.

210. Ibid., vi.

211. Blanche Wiesen Cooke, "Female Support Networks and Political Activism: Lillian Wald, Chrystal Eastman, Emma Goldman," *Chrysalis,* v. 3 (1977): 43–61, describes the close friendships of the women on Henry Street; Doris Daniels, "Lillian D. Wald: The Progressive Woman and Feminism," Ph.D. diss., City University of New York, 1976, 4–39, for description of Wald as a feminist; Dock and Stewart, *A Short History of Nursing,* 162; Lavinia Dock, "The Nurses' Settlement in New York," *Short Papers on Nursing Subjects,* (New York: M. Louise Longeway Publisher, 1900), 27–36 and reprinted in *A Lavinia Dock Reader,* ed. Janet Wilson James (New York, Garland Publishing Company, 1985), 27–36, for description of the life of the visiting nurse; Ellen Condliffe Lagemann, *A Generation of Women: Education in the Lives of Progressive Reformers,* (Cambridge, MA: Harvard University Press, 1979), 59–86, for description of Wald as progressive woman; Wald, *The House on Henry Street;* Wald, *Windows on Henry Street,* describes the pioneering work at Henry Street.

212. Lavinia Dock, "Reflections on Education for Nurses and Laity," (labeled To IMS from LLD, June 1947, Unpublished paper, p. 2), Isabel Maitland Stewart, History of Nursing, series 4, Fiche 2637, TC, CU.

213. Ibid., 2.

214. Ibid.

215. Dock, "The Nurses Settlement in New York," 31.

216. Ibid., 32.

217. Bullough and Bullough, *The Emergence of Modern Nursing,* 158, Ruth Knollmueller, "Some Beginnings and Developments in and of Significance to Public Health Nursing," (Unpublished papers), for a comparison of dates in nursing and public health nursing with other significant

events; Fitzpatrick, "A History of the National Organization for Public Health Nursing," 13.

218. Wald, *The House on Henry Street,* 27.

219. Ibid., 28; Bullough and Bullough, *The Emergence of Modern Nursing,* 158–160, describes how Wald found financial support for the Henry Street Settlement through the contributions of wealthy friends Mrs. Solomon Loeb and Jacob Schiff.

220. Nutting, "The Training of Visiting Nurses," and "The Social Services of the District Nurse," *A Sound Economic Basis For Schools of Nursing,* 112–124, 125–132; Wald, *Windows on Henry Street,* 78–9, "Twenty-Five Years of Nursing Education in Teachers College 1899–1925," 24–28; Lillian Wald, "Nurses' Settlement," *AJN,* 1 no. 1 (October 1900): 39, By 1900 Wald already used the Henry Street Settlement to give students experience in district nursing.

221. Wald, *The House on Henry Street,* 53.

222. Ibid., 51–53.

223. Fitzpatrick, "A History of the National Organization for Public Health Nursing," 13.

224. Mary S. Gardner, "The National Organization for Public Health Nursing," *Visiting Nurse Quarterly,* 4 no. 3 (July 1912): 13.

225. Adelaide Nutting, "Thirty Years of Progress in Nursing," *Proceedings of the Twenty-Ninth Annual Convention of the NLNE* (Baltimore: Williams and Wilkins, 1923), 105; Birnbach and Lewenson, *First Words,* 361. Nutting wrote, "The public health movement did not create the public health nurse, it found her at work in her district nursing the sick, watching over their families and the neighborhood, and teaching in the homes those sanitary practices, those measures of personal and home hygiene, which do much to prevent disease and promote health."

226. Wald, *Windows on Henry Street,* 72.

227. Nutting, "The Training of Visiting Nurses," in *A Sound Economic Basis for Schools of Nursing,* 112–124; Seymor, *A General History of Nursing,* 181.

228. Hamilton, "Research and Reform: Community Nursing and the Framingham Tuberculosis Project, 1914–1923," 8–13. Wald first contracted the services of the Henry Street Settlement nurses to the Metropolitan Life Insurance Company but questions were raised as to who controlled the definition of the work done by the nurses.

229. Wald, *The House on Henry Street,* 38.

230. Gardner, "The National Organization for Public Health Nursing," 13.

231. Ibid., 14.

232. Mary Gardner, "Report of the Joint Committee Appointed for Consideration of the Standardization of Visiting Nursing," *AJN,* 12 no. 11 (August, 1912): 894.

233. Ibid., 895.

234. Ibid., 896. Here is a distribution of agencies to which the letters of invitation from the joint committee were sent:

Visiting nurse associations	205
City and State boards of health and education	155
Private clubs and societies	108
Tuberculosis leagues	107
Hospitals and dispensaries	87
Business concern	38
Settlements and day nurseries	35
Churches	28
Charity organizations	27
Other organizations	19

    Additional letters were sent to:

different counties of the Pennsylvania State Board of Health where nurses worked	78
Nurses independently employed by the Metropolitan Life Insurance Company	204

235. Gardner, "The National Organization for Public Health Nursing," 16.

236. Ibid., 18.

237. Letter from Ella Phillips Crandall to John D. Rockefeller, 13 October 1914, RAC, RC, RG 1.1, Series 200, Box 121, Folder 1498, information on dues printed in pamphlet for the National Organization for Public Health Nursing and attached to letter.

238. Ibid. The NOPHN, under the presidency of Mary Gardner in 1914, asked the Rockefeller Foundation for financial support because of the difficulty in generating sufficient self-supporting funds for its activities from the membership fees; Letter from Jerome D. Greene to Gertrude W. Peabody, 10 November 1915, RAC, RC, RG 1.1, Series 200, Box 121, Folder 1498. The first request made by Crandall to Rockefeller was denied because the Rockefeller Foundation, although interested in public health, felt its contribution to public health would be made in a different way.

239. Letter from Crandall to Rockefeller, see attached printed PHNO pamphlet; Boardman, "Rural Nursing Service of the Red Cross," 937–939; Bullough and Bullough, *The Emergence of Modern Nursing,* 162; Clement, "Town and Country Nursing Service," 494–496; "Informal Statement Concerning the Object and Scope of the National Organization for Public Health Nursing and Its Relation to the Red Cross Town and Country Nursing Service," 5 November 1915, RAC, RC, RG 1.1, Series 200, Box 121, Folder 1498. Most of the concerns of public health nurses were seen in the larger urban cities. However, in response to the specific needs of rural public health nurses, Wald and the PHNO planned a program with the American Red Cross to organize and prepare trained nurses to meet the specific needs of nurses in rural community settings. A special course was established at Teachers College to be run in connection with the American Red Cross.

240. Sophia Palmer, "Report of the Fifteenth Annual Convention," *AJN,* 12 no. 11 (August 1912): 901.

241. Kalisch and Kalisch, *The Advance of American Nursing,* 293. The first nurse registration law passed in North Carolina in 1903.

3

The Formative Years: Nursing and Suffrage, 1893–1910

All questions having ultimate advancement of the profession are dependent upon united action for success.

Sophia Palmer, 1897[1]

Until we possess the ballot we shall not know when we may get up in the morning to find that all we had gained has been taken from us.

Lavinia Dock, 1907[2]

OVER TIME, NURSES in the American modern nursing movement came to support woman suffrage. Between 1893 and 1910, they developed collective power to establish nursing as a profession through activities in professional organizations. By 1910, the Superintendents' Society, the Associated Alumnae and the National Association of Colored Graduate Nurses had formed. Two professional journals, the *American Journal of Nursing* and the *Nurses' Journal of the Pacific Coast,* along with various alumnae magazines, were published monthly to inform, educate, and debate new ideas regarding professional concerns among trained nurses. The need for the organization (National Organization for Public Health Nursing) was recognized and thus formed by those trained nurses who worked in the new setting called public health. Uppermost in the minds of trained graduate nurses was the professional development of nursing; their efforts focused on nursing education, practice, and registration throughout these formative years. But nurses soon learned they had little control of these professional issues outside of their organizations. Nurses argued that the vote was essential because as women they were powerless in their professional and personal life without it. As they became convinced of this and gathered strength among themselves in the organizations established, they began to support other women in the suffrage movement.

During this formative period, trained nurses gained power and control of their work and education. Collectively they fought for nurse registration, non-payment of pupil nurses, eight-hour work days, uniform curriculums, and recreation for pupil nurses. Because trained nurses were mostly women, organizations wanted power and control of women's issues relevant to them. Most fundamental of these issues was their disenfranchisement, which rendered their profession defenseless against enemies of nursing reforms. Therefore, while all the women's issues of the early twentieth century addressed their goal of professional development, the issue of woman suffrage emerged as both a professional and a pragmatic concern: nursing's practical feminism directed its support of women's struggle for the vote. The nursing organizations in America which represented the individual woman nurse as well as the woman's profession of nursing, sanctioned suffrage as crucial to the empowerment of their members and to facilitate their access to political control of the profession's development.

Emma Maud Banfield (1870–1931), superintendent of the Polyclinic Hospital in Philadelphia and active member of the Superintendents' Society, argued at the Superintendents' Society's 1899 sixth annual convention that politicians did not appoint nurses to sit on boards of health because nurses could not vote. Trained nurses' expertise in community health behaviors rendered them obvious candidates for boards of health, which ensured the health of the community; however, their appointment to a board was deemed as "thrown away" by local politicians because nurses were women. Without woman suffrage, politicians had no reason to dispense the political favor of a board position on a nurse.[3]

Thus, trained nurses were controlled by these boards without their having any representation. The result was that nurses and their professional status were often treated capriciously. Banfield gave an example of a local board of health regulation which affected private duty nurses who worked on contagious cases in the community. While working on such a case, private duty nurses were prohibited by the board of health from riding a public conveyance as a measure to forestall the spread of disease. However, Banfield noted, this same rule did not apply to physicians who cared for the same cases.[4]

During the same session, nursing educator Adelaide Nutting described the work of Jane Addams (1860–1935) in Chicago. A leader in the settlement house movement, Addams exemplified what women were capable of and the expertise they possessed. Thus, the accomplishments of the settlement house movement reinforced the argument to include women's expertise on the various boards of health. Outraged by the exclusion of women from service on boards of health, the Superintendents' Society passed a motion which called for representation of the nursing profession on boards of health and to further promote action, formed a committee to advocate nursing members on such boards.[5]

At the same meeting of the sixth convention, Lillian Wald called on nurses to use their talents and practical training wherever possible in civic reforms. Founder of the Henry Street Nurses' Settlement in New York City, Wald listed a wide range of social reforms in which nurses were engaged: cleaning streets, improving conditions in tenement houses, advocating recreational facilities in cities, establishing kindergartens, pressing sanitary reforms for factory and tenement inspections, and urging protective legislation for children. People, she said, knew the important contribution of trained nurses to these reform efforts and supported the appointment of nurses to serve on boards which addressed these reforms. Aware of the political climate of bossism, Wald criticized the spoils system for appointments to these boards because that system excluded women from board membership. Therefore, she advocated civil service reform which would offer women an equal chance of membership. Wald urged nurses to extend their commitment beyond being good nurses so that they might employ their talents wherever possible.[6]

In their quest for control of their profession through suffrage, nursing organizations sought the shared experiences of other women's groups. Nursing's early affiliation with the National Council of Women (NCW), the International Council of Women (ICW), and with the International Council of Nurses (ICN) indicated the recognition of shared problems that nurses and other women faced. Each of these organizations advocated the rights of women, specifically equal suffrage for women throughout the world. The affiliation of the Superintendents' Society, the Associated Alumnae, and the National Association of Colored Graduate Nurses to these national and international women's associations indicated American nurses' deliberate support of woman suffrage. However, the support of woman suffrage by American nursing organizations was triggered by a compelling need to politically control the nursing profession.[7]

The American Federation of Nurses between 1901 and 1912 represented the Superintendents' Society and the Associated Alumnae in the National and International Council of Women. Although such representation was considered important to nursing, some nursing leaders felt that membership in the National Council of Women required too much time away from their own professional organizational work and preferred to support professional associations instead. Thus, a hesitancy developed as to whether women in nursing were better represented by a professional association or by broad women's groups in general.

However, the necessity of an alliance between nursing and other women's groups was a common theme raised at professional meetings. President of the Superintendents' Society and an active nursing leader in Detroit, Lystra Gretter (1858–1951), reiterated this theme when she addressed the ninth annual convention of the Superintendents' Society in September 1902. Gretter felt by virtue of its association with the national and international women's groups, American nursing was committed to the same goals as those groups. The ideas expressed in the preamble to the National Council of Women, as well as the International Council of Nurses and the International Council of Women, called for women to unite with a confederation of workers to improve conditions caused by ignorance and injustice which threatened their families and their nations. To be able to live up to the expectations of these groups, Gretter said that American nursing must take its place ". . . in the arena of the world's activities, and assume our share of responsibility."[8] Although Gretter does not explain what she meant by assuming responsibility, she firmly believed that nursing must unite with other women in their actions to improve the life of all people.[9]

American nurses soon learned that as women in the paid labor force or as citizens they confronted the issue of suffrage because they were not impervious to the world outside of the hospital. By 1906, four years after Lystra Gretter spoke of nursing's commitment to other women's groups, the proceedings of the Superintendents' Society and the Associated Alumnae and the articles in the *AJN* indicated that the intensifying campaign among women suffragists throughout America had become incorporated into the agenda of professional nursing. Identification with suffrage groups slowly became evident as nursing fought battles against long hours of work and opposition to nursing education, as well as struggling for state registration of nurses. At their ninth annual convention of the Associated Alumnae in 1906, the membership joined with the women of Rochester, New York, to establish a Susan B. Anthony memorial following the death that year of this suffrage leader.[10]

Sophia Palmer addressed the convention on behalf of the memorial to the famous woman suffragist and flyers were circulated to those present which explained the memorial. Palmer described Anthony's personal sacrifice in her support of women's education: Anthony had used her own financial resources in order to raise necessary funds to admit women to the full privileges as students at the University of Rochester.[11] Palmer also praised Anthony for contributing ". . . as much to the advancement of nurses as any other women, improving our legal status, and all those things we enjoy."[12] She encouraged all trained nurses to support financially the memorial to the woman suffragist and activist. The president of the Associated Alumnae, Annie Damer (1858–1915), expressed her hope that members would interest themselves and participate in the suffrage movement's effort for the memorial.[13]

During that same year, the *AJN* published a letter dated September 15, 1906, from the National American Woman Suffrage Association (NAWSA), signed by members of its Committee on Congressional Legislation. This letter from Kate M. Gordon (1861–1932), Annice Jeffrey Myers, and Florence Kelley (1859–1923), had been sent to more than 3,000 women's clubs, leagues, and other organizations throughout the country.[14] The Committee on Congressional Legislation called upon woman organizations to support the woman franchise, whether or not their primary goal was suffrage. Its text said that one reason for failure to gain the Constitutional right to vote was because women neglected to participate in the suffrage movement and did not express their sentiments on this issue to their legislators. The NAWSA leadership urged women to ask candidates, before elections, whether or not they supported the woman suffrage amendment, and they encouraged women to educate members of Congress regarding their position on suffrage. Moreover, the letter urged that each candidate's position, whether in support or opposition of woman suffrage, be made public in their local newspapers and the leaders of the NAWSA be notified of their positions. The suffragists believed that without women's full support, a joint resolution in Congress to allow women the right to vote would never gain the support of the needed two-thirds of the members of both houses of Congress.[15]

The publication of the letter in the nursing journal represented the profession's recognition of the woman movement's efforts to obtain suffrage. *AJN* editor Sophia Palmer acknowledged the letter's co-signer, Florence Kelley, as someone that "all nurses know for her work in the Consumer's League."[16] The editorial included Kelley's opinion that working women and children would not see any permanent improvement in their lives until equal suffrage was obtained. The editorial invited all nurses interested in the broad subject of suffrage to respond.[17]

The following year one of nursing's leading suffragists, Lavinia Dock, delivered a paper to the delegates at the tenth annual convention of the Associated Alumnae in 1907 entitled, "Some Urgent Social Claims."[18] Many more nurses read the paper when it was subsequently published in the July 1907 issue of the *AJN*. In her speech, Dock challenged nurses to go beyond the limits of their nursing profession and to look outward as women. She often felt that nurses were too focused on professional issues to be sufficiently aware of outside world events, and hence feared that for many nurses, suffrage was ". . . a far-off, abstract, uninteresting theme . . . to be avoided with disapproval, or with the indifference of the extreme specialist toward all outside of a specialty."[19]

Dock felt that the Associated Alumnae would fall short of its larger social obligation to the public if it failed to look beyond a restricted professional path. According to Dock the once revolutionary idea of woman suffrage was an idea that would soon be a reality. She worried that if nurses were too absorbed in patient care and nursing duties to see what was going on around them, they would miss the opportunity to prepare themselves for the changes that would occur when women got the vote. Dock gave a chronological history of the campaign for woman suffrage prepared by Alice Stone Blackwell (1857–1950), one of the editors of the *Women's Journal*. Dock shared this information with nurses in hopes that they would be better informed and more aware of the important struggle for suffrage throughout the world.

Dock's presentation carried the far more important message that nursing professionals should look at social and political problems and include social reform among their professional obligations. Dock advised the membership to become a "great moral force on all the great social questions of the day."[20] Among the social questions which Dock advised nurses to address were the issues of education, labor, prostitution, white slave laws, and sexual hygiene. Although, Dock said, "she was far from thinking that many of us individually can take any active or direct part"[21] in these social movements, at least trained nurses should give "intelligent sympathy and moral support,"[22] as well as some useful service and financial backing. She wanted nurses to support woman suffrage by discussing these social issues at various nursing association meetings and to write about them in their nursing journals. Nurses needed to broaden their understanding of their relationship with other workers, because, Dock warned, "those who only know their own specialty do not even know that one."[23]

The woman's vote was crucial to the resolution of these social ills and thus important for nurses to address. In an attempt to make nurses see the importance of political activity, Dock asked the Associated Alumnae, as an organization ever concerned about the public's opinion of nursing:

> . . . *how long we may as an organized society withhold our interest from these subjects and yet demand the interest and the respect of society as a whole for ourselves and our individual problems.*[24]

The discussion among the Associated Alumnae delegates that followed Lavinia Dock's paper at the tenth annual convention reflected hesitancy to endorse Dock's position on suffrage on the part of some members. Mary E.P. Davis agreed with Dock that the issue of woman suffrage was important to nurses. However, Davis warned, nursing legislation might be adversely affected politically if nursing took too strong a position in favor of suffrage. Davis suggested instead that nurses should understand and prepare themselves to become active, voting citizens when woman suffrage was eventually enacted.[25]

Another member of the Associated Alumnae who participated in the discussion of Dock's paper, Louise Croft Boyd, admitted that she "personally" did not believe in "women having the franchise."[26] However, after living and working for thirteen years in the state of Colorado, where women had the franchise, she observed that it was women's duty and privilege to exercise their vote. Nevertheless, in response to Davis's question of whether the women's vote improved the social conditions in that state, Boyd felt there was no improvement. She gave an example of a judge who recently won an election in Denver who she believed did more for the citizenry than any woman's vote. However, persuaded by those comments, Dock reminded Boyd that it was the women's votes who placed that judge in office.[27]

In 1908, the deliberation of nursing organizations reflected the individual nurse who put her professional needs over her personal needs as a woman. Focused on the advancement of the nursing profession, nurses were unsure of whether to support suffrage officially through their organization. Some nursing leaders argued that achieving woman suffrage was tantamount to achieving nursing's professional goals, but others feared adverse consequences from such support. Caution among some nurses was a result of their reliance on their profession for their livelihood. They practiced in an often hostile, conservative, male-dominated work environment. They worried that legislators would oppose state nurse registration acts if nurses supported an equal franchise for women.

Unfortunately, the year 1908 has been remembered as the year nursing refused to officially support woman suffrage.[28] Yet 1908 was also the year that an explosion of sentiment on this topic burst among the membership of the two existing nursing organizations. Nurses flexed their growing professional power to address issues which significantly impacted on their personal lives. At the Superintendents' Society convention that year, the superintendents heard arguments for equal suffrage from suffragist Margaret Doane Bigelow. Nurses at the larger Associated Alumnae convention had an opportunity to vote for an organizational resolution to support woman suffrage. Although nurses that year failed to rally enough support for such a resolution, the campaign to educate nurses on the suffrage issue and to persuade them to vote in favor of suffrage in the future began in earnest.

During the fourteenth annual convention of the Superintendents' Society convened in Cincinnati between April 22 and 24, 1908, suffrage supporter Margaret Doane Bigelow addressed the nursing group.[29] Standing before the superintendents, Bigelow urged them to support a woman's right to vote, arguing that together as women they could improve the social conditions of homes, cities, nation, and the world. Bigelow's address raised the social consciousness of these professional women whom she believed already knew of the untoward effects inadequate health care had on social conditions. Before she concluded her speech, she urged the Superintendents' Society to prepare a resolution in support of suffrage.[30]

Nursing educator and former treasurer of the Superintendents' Society, Adelaide Nutting, announced her appreciation for Bigelow's presentation and recognized that the speaker did not have sufficient time to speak. She predicted that "Dr. Bigelow has told us something which perhaps while we do not know about now or care about now, we will both know and care about before many years are over."[31] To afford more time for discussion on suffrage, Nutting moved that the Superintendents' Society plan more time at another meeting on this issue. Her motion was seconded and carried.[32]

This new alliance between the Superintendents' Society and the suffragist speaker did not go unnoticed by the press, and a report describing this event soon appeared in a newspaper article entitled, "Nurses Approve Woman's Rights." The 1908 article recounted that Bigelow had left the superintendents' convention immediately after delivering her speech but a messenger to ask her to return had been sent by the group. Her return to the conference hall prompted a "storm of applause," which Nutting optimistically interpreted as indicating that her ". . . sister nurses had appreciated the work of the suffrage movement."[33]

While members of the Superintendents' Society applauded Bigelow, those of the Associated Alumnae voted for the first time on the issue of organizational support for suffrage at their convention held that same year. President of the California State Nurses' Association Helen Parker Criswell welcomed the Associated Alumnae to San Francisco for their 1908 eleventh annual convention. Her opening address challenged the Associated Alumnae to solve problems which nursing faced in caring for the public, and she specifically urged them to think about their ideas of "the status of the twentieth century woman."[34] Criswell concluded by expressing her pleasure that the convention was held in the far west, a section which fostered independent thought and action.

During the afternoon session on Thursday, May 7, 1908, a letter from Anna Howard Shaw (1847–1919), president of the National American Woman's Suffrage Association, was read by one of the members of the Associated Alumnae. Shaw's letter demanded equal rights for men and women and she requested that the nursing membership pass the following resolution:

> Resolved, *That the Nurses' Associated Alumnae of the United States, numbering 14,000 members, as a company of patriotic workers, heartily endorse every well-directed movement which tends to emancipate the women of our land and give them their rightful place in government.*[35]

Associated Alumnae president Criswell then moved that the membership endorse that resolution. The vote on endorsement, following a discussion by those present, "lost by a large majority."[36]

Samples of remarks by members during the brief discussion prior to the vote represented different sentiments on the subject. A Miss Parson opposed the resolution and cited an example of an earlier discussion in which she had taken part where anti-suffragists in Massachusetts told how without the vote they could better influence the action of both Democratic and Republican legislators. A Miss DuBose retorted that if women could vote on their own, they would not have to rely on political influence to obtain what they wanted. Nurse Lockwood expressed the concern that seemed to be held by the majority of members that the Associated Alumnae had enough other issues with which to contend and should avoid taking a stand on suffrage.[37]

Genevieve Cooke (1869–1928), founder of the *Nurses' Journal of the Pacific Coast* and first vice-president of the Associated Alumnae (1908), argued in favor of suffrage. She asserted that the work of the suffragists had paved the way for nurses. Cooke said, "I think we would not have been the women we are today if it had not been for the suffragists."[38] She recalled that although in 1905 she had asked that the question of suffrage be tabled at an Associated Alumnae meeting, today, in 1908, she was of a different opinion.[39] An unidentified speaker said that the nursing membership had too little time to be able to decide if women should enter the political arena. Criswell responded that lack of time was an unacceptable excuse for nurses not to provide moral support for women who had done so much for nursing. She concluded that because those people who had the time worked towards equal suffrage for all women, ". . . as professional women we can no longer afford to withhold moral support."[40]

Finally, a Miss Wadley inquired if the objections to the resolution would be removed if the term "uplifting" were substituted for "emancipation." The discussion closed following Wadley's suggestion and the resolution was voted on by the Associated Alumnae delegates present at the convention. The majority of the delegates voted to defeat the suffrage resolution.[41]

Following the defeat of the suffrage resolution in San Francisco, the executive board of the Associated Alumnae met in New York City on October 30, 1908. Presiding officer Mary E.P. Davis read a letter from the National American Woman's Suffrage Association which invited a delegate from the Associated Alumnae to the National American Woman's Suffrage Association convention to be held in Buffalo, New York. Unfortunately, the timing was off and the meeting had already taken place, which rendered the matter moot; no action was taken at the meeting.[42]

Deliberation of the question of suffrage was not limited to conventions but was also addressed within the *American Journal of Nurses* and the *Nurses' Journal of the Pacific Coast* (NJPC). After the events of May 1908, the *AJN* and *NJPC* printed an increasing number of essays, letters, and comments depicting the varying degrees of political support for and against woman suffrage. Nursing's escalating debate on woman suffrage was directly attributed to the defeat of the suffrage support resolution by the Associated Alumnae in San Francisco that past year.

Reflecting the anger of many nurses, Dock protested the Associated Alumnae's suffrage support resolution vote in a letter published in the August 1908 issue of the *AJN*. There was no reason, she wrote, that nurses could not support suffrage except a selfish one because it required neither time to offer moral support nor did it cost money to give intelligent sympathy to the suffrage movement. Since nurses responded intelligently and sympathetically to other social reforms, Dock considered it "foolish to take up an almshouse propaganda and yet reject the belief that women should vote."[43] Dock closed her letter with her hopes that nurses would support woman suffrage and reconsider their ". . . hasty snapshot verdict."[44]

Another letter written by Dock appeared in the August 1908 issue of the *Nurses' Journal of the Pacific Coast*. Dock used this letter to express her chagrin and distress over the unbelievable defeat of the suffrage resolution. She had expected that this body of women would have responded "instinctively to the progressive step and intelligent idea"[45] and could not believe they voted as they had. Why, she asked, should nurses forget they were citizens? As citizens they already owed a great deal to the ". . . pioneers who have fought the women's fight."[46] Dock concluded her letter by asking "where were our Western sisters when this unfortunate vote came about?"[47] To Dock's question, the editor of the *NJPC* responded that she was "Not guilty!" and assured Dock that she hoped for better results at the 1909 convention.[48]

Lavinia Dock played a crucial role in educating American nurses to the suffrage issue not only by her letters to the various journals but through her monthly column in the *AJN,* "Foreign Department," where she informed nurses of international suffrage events. Dock reported in her *AJN* "Foreign Department" of August 1908 that 500 nurses marched in the Woman's Parade on June 13, 1908, in London under the Florence Nightingale banner. She described the respect that the crowds displayed toward these women and expressed regret that some British nurses were prohibited from marching for suffrage by their hospital employers. Dock deemed this interdiction to be an unjustifiable interference with these nurses' liberties because the loss of their jobs was threatened.[49]

In September 1908, nurse Edith Thuresson Kelly had a letter published in that month's issue of the *AJN* opposing the Associated Alumnae's suffrage resolution decision. Responding to Dock's report on the British suffrage parade, Kelly believed that among the 14,000 members in the Associated Alumnae, there must have been some nurses who would have gladly marched "in the great parade in London on June 13 under the Florence Nightingale banner. . . ."[50] Kelly registered her disbelief that the nursing profession had refused to support woman suffrage when they as nurses enjoyed the benefits of the political struggle waged by other woman workers. She asserted to her colleagues that once nurses achieved state registration, there could be no better cause for nursing societies to support other than the woman's fight for equal pay for equal work.

Following the Associated Alumnae's San Francisco convention in 1908, the official journal of the Associated Alumnae and the Superintendents' Society, the *AJN,* came under attack by some of its readers because of the journal's neutral stance on woman suffrage. Prior to 1908, few articles appeared in the journal regarding this issue and those that were published did not reflect the journal's support. The journal's stance angered some readers because they felt that the political struggle which so affected the nursing profession had been ignored by the profession's mouthpiece. To some, neutrality and omission of the subject represented a lost opportunity to educate large numbers of trained nurses on the matter; however, others praised the *AJN*'s neutral stance.

Writing in response to several letters to the editor which questioned the *AJN*'s neutral posture, editor-in-chief Sophia Palmer wrote an editorial in defense of the journal's position in the September 1908 issue. The editorial, entitled, "The Journal's Attitude on the Suffrage Question," reflected the position that the magazine was a "professional journal, devoted to the interests of nursing," and thus, "on every nursing subject it had a definite policy." However, in regard to all broad issues, the nursing journal maintained a neutral attitude; thus its neutral posture toward suffrage was the same as it was towards other broad issues. The *AJN* maintained this stance on the franchise because of the diversity of opinion among the women represented in the Associated Alumnae and the Superintendents' Society. Palmer classified *AJN* readers into three distinct groups: those who strongly supported woman suffrage, those who ardently opposed the issue, and those who maintained a moderate view on the subject. Palmer classified herself with the moderates.[51]

Suffragist Mary Bartlett Dixon (1873–1957), a 1903 graduate of the Johns Hopkins Training School, published her essay "Votes for Women" in the October 1908 issue of the *NJPC*. Contending that it was impossible for nurses not be involved in politics because as women they were involved even before they were born, Dixon concluded that no other issue or matter could be attended to until nurses were politically oriented. To justify her claim, she wrote how the health, wealth, and happiness of society and of the nursing profession relied on nursing's increasing political involvement in social reforms. Dixon stated that nurses took political action each time they professionally advocated better laws to control air, water, milk, food, and drug supplies, improved sewage disposal, better housing and factory inspections, regulation of fire escapes, saloons, prostitution, and sought better labor laws affecting men, women, and children. Moreover, Dixon felt that the regulation of the profession, their salaries, and their directories involved them with politics. And, she concluded, nurses' concerns with injustice in the world rendered their political involvement unavoidable.[52]

Dixon asked each nurse to find out what the voting law was in her state. She paraphrased the voter requirement in Maryland which included a clause that anyone over the age of twenty-one and who lived in a community for one year was eligible to vote *". . . except women, children, idiots, and criminals."*[53] Outraged, she chided the opponents of equal suffrage, that *". . . your first mistake was in educating your girls."*[54] History, Dixon argued, shows that in higher civilizations "woman has been accorded the nearest approach to an equality with man."[55] Thus, she urged nurses to reach for that higher level and demand equal suffrage for women.

Dock commented immediately following Dixon's work that it was "so shortsighted" of nurses not to "perceive that full political equality for women would make it possible for them to express themselves actively in reformative movements."[56] Dock optimistically wrote that she believed with a little study of the suffrage issue, American nurses would take their place "in the army of intelligent modern thinkers on this the most pressing of all present social reforms."[57]

The October 1908 issue of the *AJN* continued the discussion of the now infamous Associated Alumnae stand on the suffrage resolution. A recent contributor to the *NJPC*, Mary Bartlett Dixon, submitted a letter of criticism to the *AJN* which deplored the journal's neutral stand on the question of suffrage previously referred to in the *AJN*'s September issue. She argued that logically the nursing profession could not be interested in progressive social reforms and yet be neutral on the "broad questions." Dixon described her visit to her county almshouse as a representative of the Maryland State Nurses' Association.[58] During that time she observed that the only way a woman could improve the poor conditions of the almshouse was if she became a "lady visitor" and offered food and entertainment to the "inmates"; Dixon also learned that the only way to make significant changes at this institution was to be a member of the board of trustees. However, Dixon was told by what she described as a man "who knew" that no woman would ever be appointed as a trustee because "she has no vote."[59] Dixon pointed out that in the state of Maryland, women were politically placed on the same level as the inmates she had just seen.

Dixon concluded her letter to the *AJN* by asserting that while the Associated Alumnae refusing to support the suffrage resolution was a disappointment, the *AJN*'s editorial position of neutrality on the issue was an even greater one:

> *My next hope was that our magazine would present the question fairly to us, at least, but alas, I find the editorial staff is in the 'twilight zone' of neutrality and brushes this vital question carelessly aside.*[60]

Sophia Palmer, editor-in-chief and the president of the Associated Alumnae, responded to Dixon's criticism of the journal's neutrality in the same issue of the *AJN*. Palmer wrote that she too supported the suffrage resolution and also regretted the actions taken by the delegates at the San Francisco meeting. However, she stated flatly, that since the journal was the official organ of the Associated Alumnae and had been established to represent the views of that professional organization, the *AJN* could not take a pro-suffrage stand until its professional organization did so.[61]

Sophia Palmer interpreted the delegates' negative vote at the Associated Alumnae's convention to represent "either the sentiment of their home associations, or [their] doubt as to what that sentiment was." The important result of the vote in San Francisco, according to Palmer, was that it focused the attention of the nursing profession on the issue: many nurses were now forced to think about their position on suffrage. She believed that the time had come ". . . when our organizations may well devote careful, moderate, and sane consideration to the whole broad subject." Palmer saw the *AJN*'s proper role as a tool to inform nurses fairly on the question and provide a forum for expression of their ideas.[62]

A third letter to the editor entitled, "Extract From a Letter to Miss Dock," was included in that same October issue of the *AJN*. It was written by a nurse signed "E.L.F.," who was "intensely interested in the suffrage movement." E.L.F. thanked the journal for printing Dock's letter in its last edition but could not understand nurses' apathy toward the suffrage issue, especially given the difficulty that they experienced in achieving passage of state nurse registration laws. She hoped more light would be shed on the subject each year and that women would get the suffrage someday and "not by migrating to Colorado, either."[63]

In November 1908, the *AJN* published three more letters regarding the issue of women's right to suffrage. Adelaide Nutting's letter of support of woman suffrage stated her contention that the primary reason the delegates opposed the Associated Alumnae suffrage resolution was due to ignorance rather than any deep-seated feelings against woman suffrage. Thus, she urged nurses, individually and collectively in their state nurses' associations, to become educated on the matter. Nutting encouraged them to read the standard literature on the subject, including John Stuart Mill's (1806–1873), "Subjection of Women," as well as various journals including the *Reviews,* the *Contemporary,* the *Fortnightly,* the *Nineteenth Century,* and even the "staid and conservative *Atlantic Monthly,*" which had recently published articles on the woman suffrage issue. She also encouraged these nursing groups to arrange speakers to present their ideas, pro and con, at nursing meetings. Nutting, like Palmer, felt that it was time to "commend the whole matter to the most respectful and serious attention of our nursing associations."[64]

Another nurse who wrote to the journal to express disappointment with the Associated Alumnae's official stand on suffrage was Nora K. Holman. She wanted to know how the journal would feel once woman suffrage became a reality without the support of the nursing profession, and pointedly asked if they would "still remain neutral and uninterested?"[65]

In contrast nurse Louise Croft Boyd went on record in support of the San Francisco delegates' actions because suffrage was ". . . in no sense vital to the nursing profession." According to Boyd, nursing would jeopardize its chance to pass vital state nurse registration laws if it politically supported woman suffrage. She warned that men and legislators would ". . . quickly side against a nurse registration law which was pushed forward by women who were also working in favor of equal suffrage."[66]

Boyd's opposition to suffrage centered around the precarious position in which women found themselves whenever they attempted to change laws. Woman suffrage was opposed by some nurses, not on grounds that women were incapable of voting, but because they feared reprisal from legislators. Boyd's letter cautioned women not to upset the men who were in control of the political domain.

The December 1908 edition of *AJN* included two more letters which addressed the issue of suffrage. In a short letter, Lavinia Dock told of a politically prominent citizen in Wyoming who was grateful to a trained nurse for saving his wife's life. Dock recalled that when this Wyoming politician asked the trained nurse if there was anything he could do for her she replied, "'votes for the women of Wyoming.'" According to Dock, he included "the equal suffrage plank in the constitution of the newly made state and there it is to-day." Wyoming women had the vote when Wyoming was granted statehood. Dock concluded that she wished she knew the name of that nurse who "did this truly patriotic service for her country."[67]

Juxtaposed with Dock's letter was one signed by an "Eastern Delegate" who had supported the San Francisco decision. The eastern delegate maintained emphatically that suffrage was "none of our profession's business," and the negative vote in no way reflected on the woman suffrage movement. Each person was entitled to her own opinion but nurses should refrain from making a group decision. Thus, according to this Eastern Delegate, "it was to the Associated Alumnae's credit that the resolution was defeated."[68]

In the same December 1908 issue of the *AJN,* Dock continued to report to nurses in her monthly "Foreign Column" of significant events in the woman suffrage movement. Dock wrote that the executive secretary of the National Consumers' League and a person "well-known to nurses," Florence Kelley, had been appointed along with suffragist Carrie Chapman Catt (1859–1947) to "secure a monster petition of women, to be addressed to Congress, and asking for the extension of the franchise to the women of the United States by an amendment to the Constitution." Dock said that this suffrage committee projected more than one million names on this petition. Kelley had asked for volunteers and Dock invited nurses to participate in the Kelley-Catt undertaking.[69]

Throughout the next year the debate on whether nurses should support suffrage or not continued in the 1909 issues of the *AJN.* Editorials, featured columns and letters to the editor continued to explain to the nursing readership the pros and cons of woman suffrage. Reports featured in the journal's monthly column, "Nursing News and Announcements," revealed an increasing number of suffrage programs that nurse training school alumnae and state nursing associations were holding. In the first month of 1909, the New Jersey State Nurses' Association included in its report to the *AJN* that Lavinia Dock had lectured on almshouse reforms. At the meeting, Dock explained the important role nurses could have in the woman suffrage movement.[70]

The dialogue among nurses concerning the issue of woman suffrage and the dilemma of whether nurses should formally support suffrage efforts extended to journals other than the *AJN.* In January 1909, in the journal published by the California State Nurses' Association, the *Nurses' Journal of the Pacific Coast,* an editorial entitled, "Again the 'Woman Question,'" appeared which openly criticized the narrow view some nurses had taken on woman suffrage. This editorial asked why some members of the association would limit power of the Associated Alumnae by allowing it to travel through the years "as the faithful plowhorse."[71] The editorial staff asked why some nurses wear blinders which allowed them to move through life expending the least amount of mental or physical exertion required to provide themselves with food, shelter, and raiment? No one could deny as individuals or as a body of professional women that a great debt was owed Susan B. Anthony and other "far-seeing women" who worked hard to give them the "privilege to use and develop their God-given faculties."[72]

The California State Nurses' Association at first had voted against a resolution sent by the [California] Equal Suffrage Association in 1906, but passed it at their 1907 convention in Oakland. Thus, California nurses officially and openly supported the same resolution that had been defeated at the 1908 Associated Alumnae convention in San Francisco. For that reason, the editor encouraged her nursing colleagues not to despair because the defeat in 1908 was a blessing in disguise. Because of the numerous articles and discussions in alumnae magazines and at alumnae meetings, nurses were certain to become a more informed membership who would meet and vote again at the next convention in June 1909.[73]

The debate among nurses over support of suffrage continued in the first letter to appear in the January 1909 issue of the *AJN* in response to the "Eastern Delegate" whose letter appeared in the previous month. In this letter, M. Elma Dame noted that the "same age that has produced the highly trained nurse has raised the cry of suffrage for women." She argued that all laws which affected the health of men, women, and children, including those affecting tenement housing, child labor, and prostitution were of great concern to society's health; thus, such legislation should be of great concern to nurses. Regardless of diverse opinions held among nurses on suffrage, Dame considered the San Francisco resolution both "suitable and timely" for nurses to discuss.[74]

An editor's note followed Dame's letter which referred readers to the second volume of Dock's *History of Nursing* for a better understanding of the "relation between nursing and the movement for the emancipation of women."[75]

In the *AJN* February 1909 issue, readers found a series of four letters addressing the question of suffrage. The first was a short letter from "A Western Nurse" who praised the Associated Alumnae's position on suffrage and agreed with the opinion of the Eastern Delegate's earlier letter.[76]

The other three letters offered differing opinions. Ada M. Safford, a nurse from Plymouth, Michigan, began her letter by saying she was surprised and sorry there was any subject too broad or general for the journal to print. Safford continued that nurses needed access to as much information as possible to understand the issues of the day, and the *AJN* should be a chief source of such information. Moreover, Safford reminded her colleagues that when nursing associations asked other clubs to endorse the nurse registration movement, they would not want everybody to be "so 'narrow' that they would not listen to our appeal for registration . . . ." Safford further explained that nurse registration would be attainable when women had the vote, and the vote would be more attainable when there was nurse registration. Safford felt nurses needed to hear both sides of the suffrage debate and regarded the Associated Alumnae's vote as an indication of this need. Her letter concluded that a broad education was an important step toward political equality because knowledge of an issue came before its support.[77]

A third viewpoint was sent in by Bessie Louise Dickson from Princeton, New Jersey, who praised the *AJN*'s neutral attitude toward suffrage. She wrote that ". . . the subject of suffrage or political equality should have no place in a magazine devoted to *nursing* [italics hers]."[78] However, she did request the journal print a letter by President Theodore Roosevelt expressing his view on the issue. The *AJN* complied with Dickson's request: President Roosevelt's letter appeared, dated November 10, 1908. In it he stated that:

> *personally, I believe in woman suffrage, but I am not an enthusiastic advocate of it, because I do not regard it as a very important matter.*[79]

Roosevelt also asserted that neither did many women regard it as an important matter. He offered the contemporary bromide that men and women should function equally but in their separate spheres; he further described the "perfect life" as one in which man and woman were husband and wife, and the husband financially supported the family while the wife managed the home and children.[80]

Despite such conservative opposition, Dock continued to inform American nurses of international suffrage events through her "Foreign Department" column. In the March 1909 issue, she described the political deprivation of Russian women, and announced that women in Belgium and Sweden had obtained the franchise. However, in the April edition, Dock retracted her announcement of woman suffrage in Sweden and explained how the mistake had been made. From several journals and a transatlantic cable, Dock inferred that the franchise mentioned included every citizen. However, Dock acknowledged that the cable was incorrect, for only men in Sweden had the vote.[81]

Dock's commitment to enlightening nurses on the subject of woman suffrage found a willing audience among many of the local alumnae and state nursing associations. An announcement appearing in the featured "Nursing News and Announcements" in the March 1909 issue of the *AJN* related that Dock had addressed an audience of more than forty nurses of the Paterson General Hospital Alumnae Association in New Jersey on the "relation of the woman's suffrage movement to nursing" in February 1909.[82]

In the May 1909 issue of the *NJPC,* Dock continued her argument regarding the relationship between nursing and woman suffrage. Dock acknowledged that for most nurses, active participation in the woman suffrage movement was impossible because of their nursing duties. Nevertheless, Dock wanted nurses to recognize that their existence as professionals, their opportunities as individuals, and their social, educational, and economic status as women were the result of the suffrage movement. Therefore, nurses owed the suffrage movement their allegiance, loyalty, gratitude, and moral support, all of which could be given ". . . without taking time from our professional considerations." Dock defined the woman movement as the "gradual pressure of woman onward into opportunities of fuller and broader living." She reminded her readers of the first woman's rights meeting in 1848 at a time when "no means of self-support was open to refined women save only teaching, for meager pay and under repressive circumstances," when even the value of a woman's education was questioned. Dock remarked that these unjust conditions which women faced in 1848 were challenged by the pioneering woman suffragists who fought the system without even having the right to vote. Nurses were reminded that ". . . we must not forget that everything was said in opposition to the reform of nursing that is to-day said about voting." Dock invoked the founder of modern nursing to draw an analogy: Florence Nightingale, considered by Dock to be a shining star among women pioneers, a "revolutionist," and a "suffragist," used the international prestige she had earned in the Crimea to help her overcome the opposition of men in hospitals "who resented her changes." Thus, nursing reforms in hospitals, nurse education, and improved social status were the result of women pioneers who through their efforts established ties with other women pioneers of the suffrage movement. According to Dock, therefore, nursing and the woman movement were inextricably tied together.[83]

As was the custom, instructions to the delegates who would represent state alumnae associations at the twelfth annual convention of the Associated Alumnae to be held in St. Paul, Minnesota, in June 1909 appeared in the April 1909 issue of the *AJN*. A short paragraph subtitled, "The Suffrage," was included which addressed the question of whether or not a suffrage resolution would be on the agenda at the 1909 meeting. The editors of the journal suggested that, due to controversy and diversity of opinion over the issue of the suffrage, delegates should come prepared to vote according to their constituency.[84]

Committed to educating nurses on the suffrage question, the May 1909 issue of *AJN* printed an editorial which described a failed attempt to present nurses' opinions on both sides of the suffrage issue: about how they had wanted to publish a "very fine paper" entitled, "Suffrage for Women," written by a nurse who withdrew it when she learned that the journal would print it alongside one with an opposing view. Because the *AJN* was the official organ of the professional nursing organizations, the editors reaffirmed their resolve that the journal's position on the suffrage issue would remain neutral. Nevertheless, since the editors believed that suffrage was one of the most vital issues of the day about which nurses needed to be informed, they assured their readers that the journal would offer both pro- and anti-suffrage arguments as a method of educating nurses to make informed decisions. Thus, the editors explained that for these reasons, papers by Julia Ward Howe (1819–1910), suffragist and president of the New England Suffrage Association, and Lyman Abbott (1835–1922), an anti-suffragist, were printed in the May 1909 issue.[85]

Julia Ward Howe's paper, "Woman and the Suffrage: The Case for Woman Suffrage," argued for woman suffrage on the grounds of justice and expediency. Supporters continued to consider justice a long standing, fundamental argument for woman suffrage. The expediency of woman suffrage had been demonstrated by the number of positive social reforms in places that women voted, such as women's increased dignity and influence, improvement in the laws protecting the home and children, greater political influence, defeat of unqualified political candidates, broadened women's minds, increased opportunities to hold political office, and finally, closer family relationships.[86]

Lyman Abbott opposed woman suffrage in his paper, "The Assault on Womanhood," and asserted the existence of a "great silent constituency"[87] who opposed the idea of woman suffrage. Abbott cited biblical stories, tenets of organized religion, increased divorce rates, inequality between the sexes, and economic dependence of women as some of the rationales for his anti-suffragist views. Abbott contended that suffrage was a responsibility that few women wanted; if enough women did want the vote then they would have it. He remarked that only "a few shrieking suffragettes are eager for it because they have entered the fray and they want a victory."[88]

According to Abbott, suffragists were hysterical, unfeminine, and masculine "suffragettes." Although some "ambitious" and "philanthropic" women voiced their opinion that the ballot would accomplish political equality and moral and industrial reforms, most women remained silent and were not represented by the suffragists. Abbott argued that suffrage was a question of function, not equality: women and men were unequal. For example, he wrote, some men are needed in nursing; however, according to physicians, none were equal to a professional nurse who was a woman. Abbott concluded that the silent majority of women did not want to govern, or participate in government, or command by ballot, but rather wanted to fulfill their useful function as mothers of their families.[89]

That May issue of the *AJN* continued the suffrage debate in the two letters to the editors. Nurse Marion T. Brockway wrote in protest of a suggestion that the suffrage question would again be voted on at the next Associated Alumnae convention planned for the following month in St. Paul, Minnesota. She argued that while nurses as individuals could support the vote, the organization itself should not be involved.

Moreover, she asserted that an individual's personal opinion on the subject should not reflect whether she was a good nurse or good member of the association. Brockway closed by stating flatly that an endorsement of woman suffrage would be in ". . . direct opposition to our constitution and a crushing blow to the nursing profession."[90]

An opposing view appeared in a lengthy letter sent in by M. E. McCalmont, superintendent, Civil Hospital, Manila, P. I. McCalmont wrote that the Associated Alumnae's negative vote on the suffrage resolution in 1908 promoted a commonly-held belief that collectively, nurses were "the most narrow minded, self-satisfied and unprogressive of all classes of professional women." But McCalmont denied that nurses fitted that description and instead interpreted defeat of the resolution as a direct result of the delegates' lack of instruction and preparation on the issue.[91]

McCalmont asserted that the suffrage movement touched nurses more than any other of the Progressive Era. In reforms brought about by active women, the nurse stood out preeminently as the ". . . medium through which the desired results must be obtained." A nurse had the "valuable technical knowledge of her training," to reform the prisons, almshouses, and hospitals as well as in the questions of sanitation and hygiene. McCalmont argued that while all trained nurses would agree that care of the sick was part of their business, they also knew that a healthy mind, body, and soul depended on social conditions for which intelligent men and women were responsible. Once the graduate nurse became aware of the social conditions that needed to be reformed, she questioned, "is she then to concern herself with the effects [of these conditions] only, and lose entire sight of the causes?" McCalmont pointed out that new laws governing such things as pure food, milk, ice, and water had to be legislated by elected officials. Once granted the right to vote, women would vote for the needed legislation to improve social conditions adversely affecting health. McCalmont stated that the disgrace of the last convention could be wiped away by an overwhelmingly affirmative vote for support of a woman suffrage resolution at the next.[92]

Unfortunately, the support that McCalmont sought did not materialize at the June 1909 Associated Alumnae meeting. Throughout that year, nurses had been exposed to diverse opinions regarding nursing's formal support of woman suffrage. They were better informed in 1909 than they were at the 1908 Associated Alumnae convention and more prepared to consider their vote as a professional body on support of suffrage. Nevertheless, at the June 1909 convention of the American Federation of Nurses (AFN) held in St. Paul in conjunction with the Associated Alumnae and Superintendents' Society, nurses representing these three organizations failed to rally enough support to pass a suffrage resolution. Although many nurses were unhappy with this result, this was the last defeat of a resolution for support of a woman suffrage resolution by a major nursing association.

President of the American Federation of Nurses (AFN) Adelaide Nutting spoke of advancements within the modern nursing movement at the AFN's second meeting held in St. Paul.[93] Nutting described accomplishments such as the development of post-graduate work in nursing, growth of nursing practice in areas of district nursing, visiting nursing, and school nursing, programs to prevent tuberculosis, establishment of milk stations and dispensaries to prevent infant mortality, and development of social services in hospitals and dispensaries.[94]

The modern nursing movement paralleled other world movements, which included suffrage, prohibition, moral prophylaxis, and peace. Nutting told the AFN delegates that nursing was influenced by these other movements and each needed nurses' attention. Suffrage, which she considered one of the greatest movements, needed the nursing community's support. Nutting warned the nursing audience that no matter what their individual opinions and preferences might be regarding these movements, they could not afford to remain ". . . ignorant of these matters and of the issues involved in them."[95]

At the same meeting, a member of the Chicago Society of Social Hygiene, Dr. Caroline Hedger, gave a paper entitled, "Venereal Diseases and Moral Prophylaxis," which argued for woman suffrage in order to alleviate the problems of prostitution and halt the spread of venereal disease.[96] She presumed that the woman's vote would be unified and thus would remove both prostitution and its concomitant health threat to women and men. Hedger also hoped that the woman's vote would change marital laws so that a woman would have to be informed of a fiancé's venereal disease. As women and as educated professionals, trained nurses were asked to support the ballot as a means to achieve protection against sexually transmitted diseases. Hedger asked that nurses teach the public about the potential dangers associated with venereal disease. In reply, Adelaide Nutting assured Hedger that nurses supported her ideas through their membership in the Society for Social Hygiene: furthermore, many nurses shared Hedger's views "that the enfranchisement of women meant sooner or later the destruction of prostitution."[97]

At the 1909 AFN meeting, the profession of nursing had another opportunity to demonstrate support for woman rights. Dock read to the assembly a resolution called "The Enfranchisement of Women." The AFN voted on whether or not their four delegates to the International Council of Nurses would endorse woman suffrage at the 1909 International Council of Nurses congress in London. The delegates selected by the nursing organization were Annie Goodrich, Isabel Hampton Robb, Jane Delano (1858–1919), and Nancy Cadmus.[98] The record of the convention showed that following a prolonged discussion, American nurses failed to endorse woman suffrage and thus by a vote of forty-eight against and twenty-eight supporting, ". . . the American delegates were instructed to vote in the negative upon it" at the upcoming ICN meeting.[99]

Dock later described how two of the four selected ICN delegates from the AFN reacted to the AFN's decision while in attendance at the 1909 ICN meeting held in London. When the delegates to the International Congress cast their ballots, Dock recalled that:

> . . . Of these delegates one was Miss Delano and, oddly enough, at the moment when the vote was taken she happened to be asleep in her chair. The second delegate was strangely missing. The resolution was affirmed.[100]

Thus, the American delegation registered only two votes in opposition to the suffrage resolutions. However, as a consequence of those two votes, Dock said that she had to apologize everywhere she went and feared that the next American delegation would be refused entry to the following ICN meeting to be held in Germany.[101]

In 1909, the president of the Associated Alumnae, Annie Damer, addressed the issue of suffrage at the twelfth annual convention. Damer remarked to her members, numbering 15,000, that she witnessed all through their meetings feelings of "unrest among women," and heard some nurses openly "demand" the ballot. Damer believed that nurses should advocate the right to vote and should begin their campaign by paying special attention to the new recruits in the profession, the pupil nurses. As professional women, graduate nurses had an obligation to prepare nursing students to become responsible professional citizens and thus, to focus on their political education. Students in nurse training schools should learn how to be self-governing while at school. Damer argued that the knowledge gained from self-government would extend into their political work in the community when they graduated. Pupil nurses who learned how to advocate shorter working hours in training schools would be better able to argue for legislative changes for women and for child labor reforms. She spoke with passion on this subject: "When you are asked to begin work for the enfranchisement of women, begin it right at home."[102]

Following Damer's speech, Edith Baldwin Lockwood from Granby, Connecticut, addressed the Associated Alumnae attending the twelfth annual convention about nursing's long struggle to become a profession. Lockwood spoke of the problems faced in educating nurses when using the outdated apprenticeship model of training and she decried the graduation of incompetent nurses just to meet the ever increasing demand for their services.[103] In the discussion that immediately followed Lockwood's paper, Associated Alumnae president Adelaide Nutting praised Lockwood for her comprehensive and carefully written speech. Nutting emphasized in her comments Lockwood's concluding remarks which called for the "closest harmony of all nurses" to overcome the obstacles that professional nursing faced. Annie Goodrich (1866–1954) continued the discussion, commenting that "eighteen years of this struggle has made a woman suffragist of me."[104]

Suffrage was again mentioned at the Associated Alumnae convention in a paper given by Linna Richardson, associate editor of the *Nurses' Journal of the Pacific Coast* entitled, "Reasons for Central Registries and Club Houses." Establishing nursing directories for private duty nurses was the focus of Richardson's paper in which she argued that nurses should control the business of supplying nurses to the public. She said that "a profession whose mission is to save life is surely equal to the task of *self-preservation, self-government, self-support, and self-respect* (Richardson's italics)."[105]

While advocating autonomy, Richardson spoke of an interdependence with others which was needed to promote world advancement. The nursing world was responsible to humanity, and in turn, humanity would contribute to the advancement of nursing. Richardson predicted that the professions' interest in state registration and central registries would be promoted by those people whose causes the nurses supported.

The successful nurse of the future would be wise and broad-minded enough to consider "her own welfare through every advance movement that can be used for the betterment of conditions now existing." She envisioned strength in union with thousands of nurses engaged in work and similar activities that would advance the interests of the nursing profession.[106]

Richardson's vocabulary reflected a business point of view rather than the historically altruistic one associated with nursing: she applied marketing terminology to nursing services offered to and so much needed by the public. She saw nursing service as a "commodity" that relied on the delivery of "quality and quick service." If nurses could not meet this demand, then others would do so. Although Richardson had heard that nurses were not good business women, she strongly urged them to "become good business women in short order."

Richardson's business ideas extended to running alumnae and state associations as well. Each of nursing's local and state professional groups could learn how to wisely invest its money from those already in successful business ventures. Hence, nursing groups would be better able to finance and build needed clubhouses for nurses to live together, she argued. Moreover, the clubhouses built would be large enough to include other women outside of nursing, especially those in business. She felt that nurses living together with women in business would broaden the horizons of both groups.

Richardson described to the audience this nurse-financed clubhouse in all its architectural details and how it would be cared for.[107] It would include a public parlor, a general dining room for all to congregate for meals, and large apartments with provisions for small kitchenettes; each apartment would have plain furniture, a "disappearing bed," and a large closet among its furnishings. She hoped her dream that one day nurses in every city would run this kind of a home was not too far off. However, Richardson fervently believed that without woman suffrage, women had little chance of ever advancing nursing, much less owning such a home. Bluntly, she stated:

> *Ours is a woman's profession in a man's world, and we need to realize that men will take much less interest in our advancement than we take in ourselves.*[108]

Therefore, women had to take an interest in their own lives and stop relying on men to support their professional goals. Men could not be trusted for needed nursing legislation, nor should they be; thus, nurses had to see that woman suffrage was crucial for their very existence. Richardson advised nurses to unite for the good of the whole profession and for the good of all women. She argued that the "products of our hands and brains are being appropriated to overflow the already full coffers of the rich of the world."[109] She continued that nursing's existence was becoming "a problem" which would become further complicated until "women are willing to think and plan for women." Thus, she asserted that a unified effort by nurses was needed to support the drive for suffrage. Richardson concluded with a warning that if support, which seemed to some a burden now, was not forthcoming, the burden would "one day become too great for us to bear."[110]

Following the June 1909 convention, the nursing membership of the Associated Alumnae continued to debate the issue of nursing's support of woman suffrage in the July 1909 issue of the *AJN*. The first letter printed favored woman suffrage and was initialed by H.E.S., R.N. from Denver, Colorado, where women could vote since 1893. H.E.S. explained that Denver newspapers had begun to question the purity of the milk supply being delivered in their city. Undoubtedly, she believed that all women would support a bill that provided a healthier milk supply for all people, young or old. This advocate further stated that women were free to exercise their right to vote or not, based on the issue. However, she warned that those who stayed home and did not vote would be looked on as unpatriotic, as were men who stayed home and did not vote.[111]

The second letter published, "Uses of the Married Nurse," signed M.T.J., expressed concern regarding the difficult adjustment for nurses who married and who were snubbed and "sort of dropped" by members of the profession. In passing, M.T.J. wrote of her family's recent transfer to the west where "women vote and do as they please," and of her use of her nursing skills at home, at her husband's business, and occasionally at the hospital. Trying to gain a balance between her personal and professional life, this married nurse vowed, "I shall continue to cherish the love for the work and supplement it along with my home duties . . . just because I love the life of a nurse."[112]

Dock's "Foreign Column" in the August 1909 issue of the *AJN* informed America's trained nurses of resolutions passed by the International Woman Suffrage Alliance (IWSA), which represented more than a million women in London, in May, 1909. Dock wrote that ". . . we are of the opinion that no woman can afford to be ignorant of these re-markable events," and proceeded to publish the resolutions of the IWSA's quinquennial congress.[113]

In Dock's October 1909 contribution, she referred to the international woman's struggle for better education. A better education was part of a larger movement to improve the economic status of women; however, this too faced worldwide opposition. Dock predicted that nursing registration, another international woman's struggle, would not be forthcoming until women could vote. In England, nurses faced a more difficult task in obtaining registration than did American nurses because they had to secure that legislation from one deciding body, the Parliament. However, in America, if one state denied nurse registra-tion, the statute could be passed in another one.[114]

By 1910, state associations had been busy informing their member-ships of Progressive Era reform movements and some began reporting their support for woman suffrage. The Maryland State Association of Graduate Nurses included a report of its seventh annual meeting held on February 10th and 11th, 1910, in the April 1901 issue of the *AJN*. It re-ported 304 active members, all of whom had the opportunity to attend the various talks at the convention and listen to topics which covered the suppression of the white slave trade, nurse registration, work in the pre-vention of infant mortality, Red Cross work, diet in treatment of dis-ease, and information about the pure food bill. On the second day of the conference, the Maryland association heard Mrs. William M. Ellicott, president of the Equal Suffrage League, speak on the subject of municipal franchise for women in Baltimore. The notice further stated that Ellicott had won advocates to the cause, "insomuch that the association by a large majority endorsed the bill before the [Maryland] legislature."[115]

American nurses read in Dock's March 1910 column about the forced feeding of English political prisoners who were woman suffrag-ists. Several British nurses were among the prisoners force-fed. The forced feeding, which aroused worldwide concern, also provoked the medical establishment in England to protest this procedure. Dock wrote that a British nurse, a Miss Wilson, protested that taxes women paid were used to support a government that denied them the "right of representation."[116]

In Dock's April column she included a story about two Russian congresses held in St. Petersburg. One congress, run by a group of neuropathologists, passed a suffrage resolution because it wanted to alleviate psychical depression, a form of depression often caused by political disability. Woman suffrage was seen as one solution to the problem. At the second congress, the anti-alcoholic group also passed a resolution in support of suffrage. The second group said, ". . . to combat alcoholism successfully, women should be enfranchised."[117]

Throughout the year, the nursing readership responded to the strong views expressed by Lavinia Dock. Unable to secure unanimous support of suffrage within the profession, nurses nevertheless became involved in discussion of the issue. One letter reflected the dialogue incited by Dock's publicity campaign. The author of "Forced Feeding of Political Prisoners" reacted unfavorably to Dock's earlier column about the suffragists who were being forced-fed in English prisons. An English nurse, "J.B.," was outraged that some of the British prisoners were nurses. Ashamed of the behavior of her countrywomen for making such a commotion, she wrote," . . . as much as we may want the suffrage, they certainly do not assume a very ladylike manner in resisting so actively." J.B. argued that these English women jeopardized respect from men for their ideas.[118]

The May issue of the *AJN* carried Dock's rebuttal to J.B.'s letter. Dock said in her response that the hunger strike waged by the political prisoners was due to poor treatment of the imprisoned English suffragists. The usual division of criminals was violated and they received treatment afforded to common criminals rather than treatment afforded to political criminals. As a result of their resistance by means of the hunger strike, women "suffragettes" were finally, after much protest, treated as political prisoners. Moreover, Dock pointed out to J.B. that the benefits women now enjoyed were the result of the ". . . 'unladylike commotion' carried on by all those women who first broke bonds."[119]

Dock reported later in 1910 that woman suffrage was making great progress in France and that the French publication, *Bulletin professional des Infirmieres et Gardes-Malades,* had published an extensive resume of the movement.[120]

The impact of the issues broached by Dock and the *AJN* were equally crucial to the members of the National Association of Colored Graduate Nurses (NACGN). In its third year of existence in 1910, the NACGN addressed issues of injustice towards African-Americans: the education of nurses, nurse registration, and health concerns of the

African-American community. The NACGN's relation of women's issues, particularly suffrage, was indirect but nevertheless pertinent to its work. Its connection with the larger woman's movement was evident through its affiliation with the International Council of Nurses.

The minutes of the third annual meeting of the NACGN held in August 1910 included the reading of an invitation from secretary of the ICN, Lavinia Dock. The International Council of Nurses for the first time invited the National Association of Colored Graduate Nurses to send a representative to the next international conference in 1912.[121] While the minutes do not record a discussion or resolution following the reading of Dock's invitation, a subsequent letter from Dock was read at the fourth annual meeting held in Washington, D.C., in August 1911. The unpublished minutes contained references to the letter in which Dock thanked the NACGN for extending an invitation to attend its convention. In her letter Dock requested that a fraternal delegate be sent to the next ICN meeting to be held in Cologne, Germany, in August 1912, with a "full report of work done by colored graduate nurses."[122] Consequently, the NACGN's connection with the broader international community of nurses developed and a NACGN delegate attended the 1912 ICN convention. While no official support of the members of the NACGN and woman suffrage appeared in the NACGN minutes, the fact that the NACGN was invited by the International Council of Nurses and the NACGN accepted indicates that the NACGN was interested in issues affecting women and nurses, including woman suffrage.

Although the NACGN was welcomed in the international nursing community, its participation in American nursing continued to be absent from the Associated Alumnae and the Superintendents' Society. In the August 1910 issue of the *AJN,* the inter-state secretary of the Associated Alumnae, Agnes G. Deans (1871–1948), wrote of the interest state nursing associations showed in Progressive Era reform activities. However, integration of black and white nurses was not among her list of topics. During Deans's presentation to the thirteenth annual convention of the Associated Alumnae, she announced that the District of Columbia had prepared an upcoming series of lectures for members living in the District of Columbia. Deans reported that one of the lectures covered the issue of woman suffrage and was titled "An Argument for Equal Suffrage."[123] Deans also identified the most widely discussed topics at alumnae meetings around the country, which included tuberculosis, almshouse nursing, Red Cross work, central nursing directories, moral hygiene, state registration, district nursing, school nursing, social service work, the nurse in relation to public health, and nursing of the insane. Although Deans did not include woman suffrage on her list, these subjects were used by suffragists to make a case for the nursing profession's support of woman suffrage.[124]

The issue of suffrage permeated the *AJN* issues. Minnie Goodnow (1875–1952) wrote an article, "An Aroused City," for the column, "Department of Visiting Nursing and Social Welfare," in the *AJN*. At that time, Goodnow was the superintendent at Bronson Hospital, Kalamazoo, Michigan, and had observed that a "remarkable movement" had occurred in that city. Families were becoming very interested in medical knowledge and women were involved in learning ways to keep their families healthy. Goodnow believed that once women knew what influenced health, such as clean milk, pure water, and better schools, they would understand why woman suffrage was so important. She predicted that even the most conservative woman would ask for the ballot once she understood what the vote could mean to her family's health. Goodnow recalled that one "sweet, retiring mother," who had attended one of the classes where social evils were discussed finally "spoke out with a voice that thrilled with emotion, 'If these things are so, I see why women need to vote. I never did before.'"[125]

After reading Dock's book, *Hygiene and Morality,* M. E. Cameron, *AJN* editor for the featured column, "Book Reviews," wrote a review of Dock's book. Cameron described it as an outline of the medical, social, and legal aspects of venereal disease designed as a manual for nurses and lay people. In her review, Cameron supported Dock's belief that only through the ballot could women effect the "downfall of prostitution" which Dock considered one of the most important preventive measures for venereal disease. Cameron believed that the book would make any nurse undecided about supporting suffrage before reading the book, quite clear of her support after.[126]

In December 1910 *AJN* readers mourned the death of several prominent late nineteenth-century reformers, marking the end of an era. In a short editorial each person's achievement was recognized: Elizabeth Blackwell pioneered the field of medicine for women; Florence Nightingale established modern nursing; Julia Howe fought for woman suffrage; and Henri Dunant, the only man among them, founded the International Red Cross Society.[127] The nursing profession memorialized these distinguished leaders, further pointing up the awareness that nursing exhibited in regard to pioneers within the woman and modern nursing movements.

The formative years 1893–1910 closed without any official support of suffrage from American nursing organizations. Notwithstanding, while nurses focused on the issues of their daily practice, their organizations grew in size and became more effective in achieving their goals.[128] Suffrage became an issue that was discussed and deliberated by individual members as well as the organizations themselves. By 1910, the growing interest in the suffrage movement among nurses coincided with the rise of activity within the woman suffrage movement itself. The drive to obtain signatures on petitions for woman suffrage in 1908 and the leadership of Carrie Catt in the suffrage movement contributed to increasing activity among the American public in general. At the same time, nurses began to see the political gains the vote offered to the nursing profession, spurring a rise in suffrage activities of both individual nurses and professional nursing organizations.

American nurses also supported the international community of nurses, who by this time officially had supported suffrage resolutions. Professional nursing organizations formed during this period showed signs of maturity and subsequently were better able to shift their interest in suffrage from the parochial concerns of the profession to the more global concern for a healthier society.

NOTES

1. Sophia Palmer, Training School Alumnae Associations, *First and Second Annual Conventions of the American Society of Training Schools for Nurses* (Harrisburg, PA: Harrisburg Publishing Co., 1897), 55, ANHNC, TC, CU, MML, New York; Reverby, *Annual Conventions,* 55.

2. Lavinia Dock, "Some Urgent Social Claims," *AJN,* 7 no. 10 (1907): 901; Janet Wilson James, ed., *A Lavinia Dock Reader* (New York: Garland Publishing Company, 1985), 901.

3. Maud Banfield, *Sixth Annual Convention of the American Society of Superintendents of Training Schools for Nurses* (held in 1899) (Harrisburg, PA:

Harrisburg Publishing Co., 1900), 34, ANHNC, TC, CU, MML, New York.

4. Banfield, *Sixth Annual Convention of the ASSTSN* (held in 1899), 31–37.

5. Adelaide Nutting's contribution to the Discussion on Methods of the Contagious Department of the Boston City Hospital (by Miss Riddle), *Sixth Annual Convention of the ASSTSN,* 31–37.

6. Wald, "The Nurses' Settlement," *Sixth Annual Convention of the ASSTSN,* 55–57.

7. See Chapter Two, "The Associated Alumnae and the Superintendents' Society Affiliate as the American Federation of Nurses."

8. Gretter, Opening Address, *Proceedings of the Ninth Annual Convention of the ASSTSN,* 7.

9. Ibid.

10. Discussion of the Susan B. Anthony Memorial by Sophia Palmer at the Ninth Annual Convention of the NAA [September, 1906] p. 328, Unpublished proceedings, Mugar Memorial Library, Nursing Archives, American Nurses Association, Board of Directors Minutes: 1897–1949 (Records of Associated Alumnae of U.S. and Canada, 1897–1912), N 87, Box 33, Boston University, Boston (hereafter cited as MML-NA); and in Sophia Palmer, Discussion of the Susan B. Anthony memorial, Proceedings of the Ninth Annual Convention of the NAA, *AJN,* 6 no. 10 (1906): 763; Finch, *Carey Thomas of Bryn Mawr,* 248, refers to a Susan B. Anthony fund established following Anthony's death in 1906 for the purpose of raising funds for equal suffrage.

11. Rheta Childe Dorr, *Susan B. Anthony: The Woman Who Changed the Mind of a Nation* (New York: Frederick Stokes Company, 1928), 337–339. Anthony had wanted the University of Rochester to become coeducational and successfully raised the funds needed to do so; she pledged her life insurance premium to complete the funding needed for the coeducational fund to convince the university trustees to admit women.

12. Discussion of Susan B. Anthony Memorial [September, 1906] p. 328, Unpublished proceedings, MML-NA, N 87, Box 33; and Palmer, "Discussion of the Susan B. Anthony memorial," *Proceedings of the Ninth Annual Convention of the NAA,* 763.

13. Discussion of Susan B. Anthony Memorial [September, 1906] p. 327–328. Unpublished proceedings, MML-NA, N 87, Box 33; Discussion of the Susan B. Anthony memorial, *AJN,* 762–763.

14. Editorial Comment, "The Equal Suffrage Policy," *AJN,* 7 no. 1 (October 1906): 7.

15. Letters to the Editor, "Equal Suffrage Movement," *AJN*, 7 no. 1 (October 1906): 47–48.

16. "The Equal Suffrage Policy," *AJN*, 7.

17. Sophia Palmer, Editorial Comment, "The Equal Suffrage Policy," *AJN*, 7, no. 1 (October 1906): 7.

18. Dock, "Some Urgent Social Claims," 895–901; James, *A Lavinia Dock Reader*, 895–901.

19. Dock, "Some Urgent Social Claims," 894; James, *A Lavinia Dock Reader*, 894.

20. Dock, "Some Urgent Social Claims," 899.

21. Ibid.

22. Ibid.

23. Ibid.

24. Ibid.

25. Mary E.P. Davis, The Tenth Annual Convention of the NAA discussion of paper, "Some Urgent Social Claims," *AJN*, 7 no 10. (July 1907): 901–903; James, *Lavinia Dock Reader*, 901–903.

26. Louise Croft Boyd, The Tenth Annual Convention of the NAA discussion of paper, "Some Urgent Social Claims," *AJN*, 7 no. 10 (July 1907): 901–903; James, *Lavinia Dock Reader*, 901–903.

27. Boyd, ibid.

28. Very often historians use 1908 as a reference for when nursing vetoed a suffrage amendment at the Associated Alumnae Annual Convention in San Francisco.

29. Margaret Doane Bigelow, Letter from the Ohio Woman Suffrage Association, *Proceedings of the Fourteenth Annual Convention of the ASSTSN* (Baltimore: J.H. Furst, 1908), 87.

30. Margaret Doane Bigelow, Address by representative from National Woman's Suffrage Association, *Proceedings of the Fourteenth Annual Convention of the ASSTSN* (Baltimore: J.H. Furst, 1908), 122–124.

31. Adelaide Nutting, Discussion of Address by representative from National Woman's Suffrage Association, *Proceedings of the Fourteenth Annual Convention of the ASSTSN* (Baltimore: J.H. Furst, 1908), 124–125.

32. Nutting, ibid.

33. "Nurses Approve Woman's Rights," (name of newspaper and date not recorded), 1908, p. 108. HMD-NLM, NLN-MS. C. 274, Box 6, Bethesda, MD.

34. Helen Parker Criswell, "Address of Welcome to the NAA, May 5, 1908," *Nurses' Journal of the Pacific Coast (NJPC)*, 4 no. 6 (June 1908): 254.

35. Report of the Eleventh Annual Convention of the NAA, A Letter from Mrs. Shaw, *AJN*, 8 no. 10 (July 1908): 860. Shaw was reported as the president of the Woman's Suffrage League.

36. Report of the Eleventh Annual Convention of the NAA, A Letter from Mrs. Shaw, 860; Helen Parker Criswell, Discussion of the suffrage resolution, Eleventh Annual Convention of the NAA, 1908, p. 70, Unpublished proceedings, MML-NA, N 87, Convention Proceedings, Box 12, Folder 1. The discussion preceding the vote was not included in the published minutes but was found in the unpublished proceedings.

37. Discussion of the suffrage resolution, Eleventh Annual Convention of the NAA, 1908, pp. 70–72, Unpublished proceedings, MML-NA, Convention Proceedings, Box 12, Folder 1. Nurses were identified without their first names. Miss Parsons may be Sara Elizabeth Parsons (1864–1949), president of the NLNE in 1916.

38. Genevieve Cooke, Discussion of the suffrage resolution, Eleventh Annual Convention of the NAA, 1908, p. 70, Unpublished proceedings, MML-NA N87, Convention proceedings, Box 12, Folder 1.

39. Although mention of a resolution or question of suffrage in 1905 was referred to, no records in the published or unpublished material have been found.

40. Criswell, Discussion of the suffrage resolution, Eleventh Annual Convention of the NAA, p. 72.

41. Discussion of the suffrage resolution, Eleventh Annual Convention of the NAA, p. 72.

42. Invitation to send delegate to the National [American] Woman's Suffrage Association: read at the executive board meeting of the NAA on October 30, 1908, p. 115, Unpublished minutes, MML-NA, N87, Board of Directors Minutes: 1897–1949 (Records of Associated Alumnae of U.S. and Canada, 1897–1912), Box 33.

43. Lavinia L. Dock, "The Suffrage Question," *AJN* 8 no. 11 (August 1908): 926.

44. Ibid.

45. Lavinia L. Dock, The Letter Box, *NJPC*, 4 no. 8 (August 1908): 366.

46. Ibid.

47. Ibid.

48. There is no record of the NAA voting on another resolution in 1909.

49. Lavinia Dock, Foreign Department: "Items," *AJN*, 8 no. 11 (August 1908): 914–915.

50. Edith Thuresson Kelly, "Letters to the Editor, A Protest," *AJN*, 8 no. 12 (September 1908): 1003. In the letter Edith Thuresson Kelly identified herself as a nurse when she wrote ". . . we as nurses . . . ."

51. Editorial Comment, "The Journal's Attitude on the Suffrage Question," *AJN*, 8 no. 12 (September 1908): 956.

52. Mary B. Dixon, "Votes for Women," *NJPC*, 4 (October, 1908): 443; Stevens, *Jailed for Freedom*, 193, 202. Stevens mentions and includes photograph of Mary B. Dixon among the militant suffragists associated with Alice Paul. *Johns Hopkins Nursing Alumnae Directory*, (Baltimore, MD: Development and Alumnae Services, Johns Hopkins University), 136.

53. Dixon, ibid., 443.

54. Dixon, ibid.

55. Dixon, ibid., 447.

56. Lavinia Dock, comment following Mary Dixon, "Votes for Women," *NJPC*, 4 (October, 1908): 447.

57. Dock, ibid., 447.

58. The letter indicated that Dixon resided in Easton, Maryland so the presumption is the almshouse was located somewhere in that county.

59. Mary B. Dixon, Letter to the Editor, "A Criticism of the Editor." *AJN*, 9 no. 1 (1908): 49.

60. Dixon, ibid.

61. Sophia Palmer, "Editorial policy explained," *AJN*, 9 no. 1, (October 1908): 49–50.

62. Palmer, ibid., 50.

63. E.L.F., Letters to the editor, "Extract From a Letter to Miss Dock," *AJN*, 9 no. 1 (October 1908): 50–51.

64. Adelaide Nutting, Letters to the Editor, "The Suffrage," *AJN*, 9 no. 2 (November 1908): 135.

65. Nora K. Holman, Letters to the Editor, "The Suffrage," *AJN*, 9 no. 2 (November 1908): 135.

66. Louise Croft Boyd, Letters to the Editor, "The Suffrage, Another View," *AJN*, 9 no. 2 (November 1908): 136.

67. Lavinia L. Dock, Letters to the Editor: "A Nurse's Influence," *AJN*, 9 no. 3 (December 1908): 202. Dock said that she had just heard the story from one of the leaders in the suffrage movement.

68. An Eastern Delegate, Letters to the Editor, "The Suffrage," *AJN*, 9 no. 3 (December 1908): 204.

69. Lavinia Dock, Foreign Department, *AJN*, 9 no. 3 (December 1908): 199; Louise C. Wade, "Florence Kelley," in *Notable American Women*,

II: 316–19; Flexner, *Century of Struggle*, 215–16. Kelly also held the position of vice-president of the National American Woman Suffrage Association and had lived at Jane Addams' Hull House in Chicago and subsequently at Lillian Wald's Henry Street Settlement in New York.

70. Helen Stephen, Nursing News and Announcements, "New Jersey" *AJN*, 9 no. 4 (January 1909): 293–294.

71. "Again the 'Woman Question.'" *NJPC*, 5 no. 1 (January 1909): 2.

72. Ibid., 3.

73. Ibid., 4.

74. M. Elma Dame, Letters to the Editor, "The Suffrage," *AJN*, 9 no. 4 (January, 1909): 284.

75. Short note following M. Elma Dame's letter, ed., Letters to the Editor, *AJN* 9 no. 4 (January 1909): 285.

76. A Western Nurse, Letters to the Editor: Reorganization Endorsed, *AJN*, 9 no. 5 (February 1909): 359.

77. Ada M. Safford, Letters to the Editor: "The Suffrage I," *AJN*, 9 no. 5 (February 1909): 360.

78. Bessie Louise Dickson, Letters to the Editor: "The Suffrage II," *AJN* 9 no. 5 (February 1909): 360–361.

79. Theodore Roosevelt, Letters to the Editor, "President Roosevelt's Letter," *AJN*, 9 no. 5 (February, 1909): 361.

80. Ibid.

81. Lavinia L. Dock, The Foreign Department, "Items," *AJN*, 9 no. 6 (March 1909): 430–431, for the first announcement; Lavinia L. Dock, The Foreign Department, *AJN*, 9 no. 7 (April 1909): 508–511, for the retraction.

82. Nursing News and Announcements, "New Jersey: The Alumnae Association of the Paterson General Hospital," *AJN*, 9 no. 6 (March 1909): 441.

83. Lavinia L. Dock, "The Relation of the Nursing Profession to the Woman Movement." *NJPC*, 5 no. 5 (May 1909): 197–201.

84. Editorial Comment, "Instructions to the Delegates: The Suffrage," *AJN*, 9 no. 7 (April 1909): 468.

85. Editorial Comment, "The Suffrage," *AJN*, 9 no. 8 (May 1909): 547. Both papers were reported to have been originally published in the noted anti-suffragist magazine, *The Outlook*.

86. Julia Ward Howe, "Woman and the Suffrage: The Case for Woman Suffrage." *AJN*, 9 no. 8 (May 1909): 559–566.

87. Lyman Abbott, "The Assault on Womanhood," *AJN*, 9 no. 8 (May 1909): 566.

88. Ibid., 572.

89. Ibid., 573.

90. Marion T. Brockway, Letters to the Editor, "The Suffrage I," *AJN*, 9 no. 8 (May 1909): 595. In her letter Brockway referred to the New York State Nurses' Association which leads me to believe that Brockway was from New York State.

91. M. E. McCalmont, Letters to the Editor, "The Suffrage II," *AJN*, 9 no. 8 (May, 1909): 595.

92. Ibid., 597.

93. The Superintendents' Society, the Associated Alumnae, and the American Federation of Nurses held joint sessions during the first week of June in St. Paul, Minnesota. It was the Superintendents' Society's fifteenth annual meeting, the Associated Alumnae's twelfth annual meeting, and the American Federation of Nurses' second meeting (its first meeting was held in 1905).

94. Adelaide Nutting, President's Opening Remarks at the Second Meeting of the AFN, *Fifteenth Annual Report of ASSTN including Report of the Second Meeting of the AFN: 1909* (Baltimore: J.H. Furst, 1910), 101–108.

95. Nutting, ibid., 106.

96. Lavinia L. Dock, *Hygiene and Morality: A Manual for Nurses and Others, Giving an Outline of the Medical, Social, and Legal Aspects of Venereal Disease* (New York: G.P. Putnam's Sons, 1910), 90-1; and reprinted in James, *A Lavinia Dock Reader*, 90-1. Moral prophylaxis related to the self-regulation of one's moral code that inhibited sexual activity outside of marriage for men and women; this was expected to stop the spread of venereal diseases and reduce prostitution. James included a note in the front of Dock's reprinted book where James defined social hygiene as a "euphemism for VD prevention" and morality as "abolition of prostitution."

97. Caroline Hedger, "Venereal Diseases and Moral Prophylaxis," *Proceedings of the Fifteenth Annual Convention of the ASSTSN*, 147–154; Nutting, Discussion of paper: Venereal Diseases and Moral Prophylaxis, *Proceedings of the Fifteenth Annual Convention of the ASSTSN*, 154.

98. Nancy Cadmus may have been the superintendent of the Manhattan Maternity and Dispensary of New York City and a member of the Nurse Board of Examiners of the state. However, this identification has not been confirmed.

99. *Fifteenth Annual Report of ASSTSN*, 215.

100. Lavinia L. Dock, "Our Debt to the Woman Movement," *The I.C.N.,* 4 no. 3 (July 1929): 198, MML-NA, ANA N87, Box 216, Envelope 2.

101. Lavinia L. Dock, Report of the Thirteenth Annual Convention: Miss Dock Reports on the International Congress, *AJN,* 10 no. 11 (August 1910): 880; and Dock, "Our Debt to the Woman Movement," 195–199.

102. Annie Damer, "Presidential Address," Twelfth Annual Convention of the NAA, *AJN,* 9 no. 12 (September 1909): 904.

103. Edith Baldwin Lockwood, "The Limitations of the Nursing Profession," *AJN,* 9 no. 12 (September 1909): 62.

104. Annie Goodrich, Discussion following "The Limitations of the Nursing Profession" in the Report of the Twelfth Annual Convention of the NAA, *AJN,* 9 no. 12 (September 1909): 946.

105. Linna Richardson, "Reasons for Central Registries and Club Houses, Proceedings of the Twelfth Annual Convention of the ANA, *AJN,* 9 no. 12 (September, 1909): 983.

106. Ibid., 984.

107. Ibid., 985.

108. Ibid., 986.

109. Ibid.

110. Ibid.

111. H.E.S., Letters to the Editor, "The Mercenary Nurse," *AJN,* 9 no. 10 (July 1909): 760; Ida Husted Harper, ed., *The History of Woman Suffrage,* vol. 6, (New York, National American Woman Suffrage Association, 1922; New York, Arno & the New York Times, 1969), 59–67. In 1893 Colorado became the second state in the union to grant woman suffrage equal to that of men. However, equal suffrage was legislated by Colorado state law and not by constitutional amendment.

112. M.T.J., Letters to the Editor, "Uses of the Married Nurse, *AJN,* 9 no. 10 (July 1909): 761–762. This letter reflects one professional woman's dilemma when she married. Perhaps being in a suffrage state prompted M.T.J. to examine this dilemma more closely.

113. Lavinia L. Dock, The Foreign Department, "The Progress of Women," *AJN,* 9 no. 11 (August 1909): 842.

114. Lavinia L. Dock, The Foreign Department, "Letter from England," *AJN,* 10 no. 1 (October 1909): 38–41.

115. Nursing News and Announcements, "Maryland," *AJN,* 10 no. 7 (April 1910): 517; Sarah F. Martin, R.N., was the secretary of the Maryland State Association of Graduate Nurses who submitted the announcement.

116. Lavinia L. Dock, Foreign Department, "Forcible Feeding in English Prisons," *AJN*, 10 no. 6 (March 1910): 408.

117. Lavinia L. Dock, Foreign Department, "Items," *AJN*, 10 no. 7 (April, 1910): 493.

118. J.B., Letters to the Editor, "Forced Feeding of Political Prisoners," *AJN*, 10 no. 7 (April 1910): 502–507.

119. Lavinia L. Dock, Letter to the Editor, "Forced Feeding of Political Prisoners," *AJN*, 10 no. 8 (May 1909): 594.

120. Lavinia L. Dock, Foreign Department, "*Jus Suffrage* Says," *AJN*, 11 no. 2 (November 1910): 111.

121. Dock to Bradley, Invitation to attend the ICN, Third Annual Convention of the NACGN, August 18, 1910, p. 34, Unpublished proceedings, NACGNR, Schomburg, Box 1, Volume 1, New York.

122. Invitation to attend the International Council of Nurses' fourth annual convention of the NACGN, p. 37, Unpublished proceedings, Schomburg, NACGN, Box 1, Volume 1. The second letter was read by Miss Watkins at the fourth annual meeting of the NACGN.

123. The inter-state secretary was an office created in 1906 and served the purpose of reporting on the activities of the various societies within the association. Agnes G. Deans (1910), Proceedings of the Thirteenth Annual Convention of the NAA report of the Inter-State Secretary, *AJN*, 10 no. 11 (August 1910): 861.

124. Agnes G. Deans, Proceedings of the Thirteenth Annual Convention of the NAA report of the Inter-State Secretary, *AJN*, 10 no. 11 (August 1910): 861–866.

125. Minnie Goodnow, Department of Visiting Nursing and Social Welfare, "An Aroused City," *AJN*, 10 no. 9 (June 1910): 670.

126. M. E. Cameron, Book Reviews:, "Hygiene and Morality," *AJN*, 10 no. 12 (1910): 999–1001; Dock, *Hygiene and Morality*, 158-9.

127. Editorial Comment, "Death of Prominent Reformers," *AJN*, 11 no. 3 (December 1910): 159–160.

128. Deans, Proceedings of the Thirteenth Annual Convention of the NAA report of the Inter-State Secretary, 861–866. Deans reported a rise in the Association's membership between 1906 and 1910, noting that the Association's Alumnae had increased from 122 societies which represented 8,500 nurses, to 182 societies which represented 14,997 nurses.

4

The Expanding Years: Nursing Supports Suffrage, 1911–1920

Men can praise us and write poems to our eyelids, but as long as they keep the ballot away from us we are counted inferior.[1]

Catharine Waugh McCulloch, 1912

IN THE BOOK *Century of Struggle: The Woman's Rights Movement in the United States,* the author, Eleanor Flexner, depicts the period between 1896 and 1910 as a quiet time within the American woman's suffrage campaign and one that suffragists referred to as "the doldrums." While the suffrage movement experienced the doldrums, the nursing profession between 1896 and 1910 experienced a flurry of activity forming nursing organizations and developing a profession. Nursing directed its political energies toward internal professional goals rather than the more global issue of woman suffrage. After 1910, the woman suffrage campaign gained increasing strength among supporters. Concurrently, American nurses, through the newly formed state and national nursing associations, expanded their political horizons and increased their activities in order to control the profession's development. The Superintendents' Society and the Nurses' Alumnae Association were by this time well established national nursing organizations, and thus better able to concentrate on external factors which influenced the profession than they were prior to 1910. Since nursing's primary political goal centered on supporting state nurse registration acts, acquiring the vote would provide nurses with their own political voice in achieving state registration.

Nurses needed the vote in order to control legislation affecting nursing practice and education.

Nursing suffragist and secretary of the International Council of Nurses, Lavinia Dock, is among the many notable professional women who contributed to the intensifying political campaign of suffrage.[2] Influenced by the accelerated campaign and by Dock's efforts, nursing organizations between 1911 and 1920 supported woman suffrage. The profession's leadership urged nurses to study the suffrage issue so they could make informed choices regarding its support. Successful in supplying nurses with the needed information about suffrage, the American Society of Superintendents of Training Schools of Nursing (hereafter called the National League of Nursing Education [NLNE]) and the Nurses' Alumnae Association of the United States and Canada (hereafter called the American Nurses Association [ANA]) voted at their respective annual conventions to support woman suffrage. Nursing's allegiance to women's rights surfaced again and again in the many speeches, affirmed resolutions, and journal articles that addressed suffrage. Further corroboration of nursing's support of suffrage can be drawn from nursing's participation and alliance with the international nursing community and other women's organizations which openly advocated woman suffrage.

The National Association of Colored Graduate Nurses (NACGN), newly formed in 1908 and set apart from the other three nursing organizations because of racial barriers, focused its attention on several professional issues other than suffrage. Advancing nurse education, nurse directories, pay equity, and nurse registration required much of the organization's time. Yet the NACGN, like the other nursing organizations, can be viewed as supportive of woman suffrage by its affiliation with the international women's community.

The National Organization for Public Health Nursing (NOPHN), which formed in 1912, supported woman suffrage by joint resolutions with the NLNE and the ANA.

First Years after the "Doldrums"

In 1911, Lavinia Dock withdrew from the Superintendents' Society because she wanted to focus all of her attention on woman suffrage.

Friends in the Superintendents' Society recognized Dock's "long and invaluable service," and voted to retain her as an active life member.[3] Dock's influence in nursing circles continued to be strong, not only because of her long-standing friendships, but also because of her numerous articles and letters published in nursing journals.

As Dock concentrated on woman suffrage and wrote extensively on the subject, The American Journal of Nursing *(AJN)* devoted considerable space to this topic. Believing that nurses should be informed, the journal gave suffrage ". . . a hearing on both sides." As an editorial comment in October 1911 explicitly stated, suffrage was "one of the burning questions of the day and no one has a right to be indifferent . . . ."[4]

As a result of this policy, a reprint from the September 2, 1911, issue of a *Woman's Journal* entitled, "The Reason Why," by novelist Mary Johnston (1870–1936), appeared in October's issue of the *AJN*. Johnston believed that women should be granted political rights that for too long had been withheld. Without the vote, the 25 million women in this country, of whom more than 5 million worked, were unfairly represented in government. In direct opposition to the basic tenets of America, women were taxed without representation and governed without consent. Outraged, Johnston wrote that women continued to be listed among those ineligible to vote, which included children, aliens, idiots, lunatics, and criminals. She called for a change in this political travesty and the successful passage of woman suffrage.[5]

Lavinia Dock, as always, kept the *AJN*'s readership abreast of international suffrage campaigns. In September 1911 she wrote of how English nurses joined in the June 17th suffrage parade attended by well over 40,000 women. More than 200 nurses marched in their uniforms, receiving "hearty cheers" from the crowds, while other nurses marched in different groups.[6]

In a later column, Dock wrote that many more women had joined the "march of women toward enfranchisement . . . ."[7] She linked women's health care needs to political expediency, arguing that the state needed the nurses' vote. Quoting directly from the *British Journal of Nursing,* Dock concluded her column with the following:

Seeing then that every race, class, and sex is dependent in time of sickness upon skilled nursing . . . and seeing that trained nursing is intimately bound up with the health and life, and . . . the comfort and happiness of the nation; putting aside for the moment the question of justice, does it not appear that the state needs the nurses' vote?[8]

Conversely, nurses needed the states' support to pass nursing registration acts. Such acts would safeguard the public from ill-prepared nurses and protect it from anyone who simply decided to call themselves a nurse. Only trained graduate nurses would qualify for nursing registration; hence, the professional position of the graduate trained nurse would be protected.

The *AJN* printed a column called "Nursing News and Announcements" (hereafter referred to as "Nursing News"), which contained reports sent in by state and local nursing alumnae associations throughout the country. In 1911, several announcements signified a growing interest in women's rights and nursing's affiliations with other women's groups.

From Seattle, Washington, the Kings County Association of Graduate Nurses reported that it encouraged nurses to attend a pre-legislative institute along with other women of Seattle. Nurses in the state of Washington believed it was important for women to learn the "duties of citizens," since women in their state had been granted the right to vote in 1909.[9]

The Maryland State Association of Graduate Nurses announced that it had fulfilled the initial purpose of the association with the successful passage of Maryland's state nursing registration laws. However, during the struggle for state registration, the Maryland Association had widened its "field of influence" through affiliation with the Federation of Women's Clubs. The Maryland State Nurses' Association had worked together with the Infant Mortality Congress and endorsed white slave and pure food bills, established a central nursing registry, and had supported "the municipal suffrage movement."[10]

In March 1911 in the *AJN,* the Graduate Nurses' Association of Virginia announced that suffragist author Mary Johnston had given a lecture entitled "Equal Suffrage" during its eleventh annual meeting. The president of the state Suffrage League of Richmond, B. B. Valentine (1865–1921), was listed among the participants of the program.[11] Edna Foley (1879–1943), leader of the Chicago Visiting Nurse Association, wrote of Mary Johnston's suffrage address in the *AJN's* monthly column, "Visiting Nurse and Social Welfare." Johnston had spoken of the rapidly growing Virginia Equal Suffrage League and how many trained nurses stood among its members. She referred to the list of nursing members which included Agnes Randolph, president of the Virginia State Associ-ation of Nurses and great-granddaughter of Thomas Jefferson.[12]

As secretary of the International Council of Nurses (ICN) Lavinia Dock included an announcement in the featured column "Nursing News" in the October 1911 issue of the *AJN*. Dock informed nurses of three resolutions that would be voted on at the Congress of Nurses to be held in Cologne, Germany, in August 1912. The international reso-lutions highlighted the state's need to support central nursing issues such as the care of old and infirm nurses, the endorsement of state reg-istration, the improvement of educational standards, and recognition of the importance the women's vote had in shaping "a more just social order."[13] Although Dock advised the ANA's state associations to study all of these issues, she wanted special attention paid to woman suffrage. Dock hoped that delegates sent to represent the state associations at the annual ANA convention would be given "explicit instructions" concern-ing woman suffrage. In this way, when the state delegates voted for the ANA's four candidates to attend the ICN meeting in Cologne, Germany, the majority opinion of the ANA membership would be represented. Dock wanted to avoid the dilemma experienced by the four poorly in-structed American delegates at the ICN conference held in London the previous year. This time, she wanted the international nursing delegates to be given a clear message as to whether or not American nursing sup-ported the international woman suffrage resolution.

Indiana nurses contributed an announcement to the November 1911 issue of *AJN*, reporting that Sophia Palmer, editor-in-chief of the *AJN*, spoke in favor of woman suffrage while at the Indiana State Nurses' Association ninth annual convention. In her address, Palmer described the difficulty experienced by nursing when establishing nurse-operated registries. In light of the resistance, Palmer spoke of ". . . her conversion to suffrage."[14]

Although excluded from the other national nursing organizations, the National Association of Colored Graduate Nurses (NACGN) par-ticipated in activities of the International Council of Nurses (ICN). Leaders in the NACGN corresponded with the ICN, sent delegations to international meetings, and included delegation reports at NACGN meetings. In doing so, the NACGN united with the international community of nurses and women in its drive for woman suffrage. At the fourth annual meeting of the NACGN held in 1911, one of its members read a letter from the secretary of the ICN, Lavinia Dock. In her letter, Dock thanked the NACGN for inviting her to attend one of their annual meetings. In turn, Dock invited the NACGN to send another delegate to the 1912 International Council of Nurses to be held in Cologne, Germany. The NACGN acted on her request and selected Rosa Williams to be the NACGN delegate.[15] At the NACGN convention the following year, Williams read her account of the 1912 ICN meeting in Germany. However, there was no mention of suffrage in her report.[16]

The public activity of women throughout the United States in 1912 was "greater" than ever before. As more states granted women full suffrage rights, it seemed to some that woman suffrage was "destined to prevail."[17] That same year woman suffrage gained nursing's official approval. The ANA sent its four delegates to the ICN prepared to support an international woman suffrage resolution, which passed. State and local alumnae nursing associations studied the issue of woman's rights by engaging suffrage speakers and affiliating with other women's groups interested in social reform.

The *AJN* continued to print announcements that reflected nursing's interest in suffrage throughout 1912. The Philadelphia General Hospital Alumnae Association reported in the March 1912 issue of the *AJN* on its recently held successful woman suffrage program. One of the suffrage speakers, Mrs. Rudolph Blankenberg, spoke of women's accomplishments and asked the group to support woman suffrage and "civic righteousness." The second speaker, Mrs. Lawrence Lewis, Jr., represented the Equal Franchise Society and encouraged nursing alumnae members to join.[18]

Lavinia Dock continued to use her monthly column in the *AJN* to educate nursing readers on woman suffrage and to influence their opinions. In the April 1912 issue, Dock again urged state nursing associations to prepare their delegates to vote on a suffrage resolution at the ANA's annual convention in June of that year. Dock wrote in the April issue as she had in the October 1911 issue that she believed a clear directive from American nurses on woman suffrage needed to be given to the American delegates who would attend and vote on an international suffrage resolution at the ICN meeting to be held later that year in Cologne, Germany.[19]

Dock's timely request to the nursing associations seemed to be effective in many instances. Nursing's movement towards support of woman suffrage became increasingly more apparent as state associations announced meetings held on the subject and resolutions passed in support of suffrage. The Graduate Nurses' Association of Virginia held its twelfth annual meeting in Lynchburg in March of 1912. At the meeting, following two "impassioned appeals to nurses" presented by Mrs. John H. Lewis, president of the Equal Suffrage League in Lynchburg, and Lila Meade (Mrs. B. B.) Valentine, president of the Equal Suffrage League in Virginia, the nursing membership supported a woman suffrage resolution:

> *Resolved that the Graduate Nurses' Association of Virginia endorse the principle of Equal Suffrage for men and women as the most effective means of securing equal privileges and opportunities in the legal, industrial and professional world, and for the promotion of the physical, mental and moral health of all the people.*[20]

The resolution passed by a large majority with no opposition registered and only a few abstentions.[21]

Indiana nurses announced their support of woman suffrage in the May 1912 issue of the *AJN*. The Indiana State Society of Superintendents of Training Schools for Nurses had invited professor of household economics at Purdue University, Henrietta Calvin, to speak on woman suffrage. In addition, the announcement noted that the Indiana State Nurses' Association, at their ninth semi-annual convention, had agreed to endorse woman suffrage at the next national convention planned for June of that year.[22]

While American nurses considered their professional suffrage stands, Dock supplied them with information about their English colleagues. Nurses read in the May 1912 issue of the *AJN* of the struggle English women and nurses faced in obtaining woman suffrage and state registration. Dock reported that the National Council of Nurses from Great Britain and Ireland had already supported woman suffrage and planned to extend its endorsement to the international suffrage resolution at the ICN meeting in Cologne, Germany. She wrote about the six English nurses who were among those "suffering imprisonment and hard labor in the cause of setting women free . . . ."[23] Dock used her story to reaffirm the political link between nursing's support of woman suffrage and the successful attainment of state nurses' registration.

At the Superintendents' Society's eighteenth annual convention held June 3–5, 1912, professor at the University of Chicago School of Civics and Philanthropy, lawyer, vice-president of the National American Woman Suffrage Association, and president of the Woman's City Club, Sophonisba Preston Breckinridge (1866–1948), welcomed the superintendents to Chicago. Breckinridge opened the convention by praising the advances in nursing education made by the Superintendents' Society, and commending its professional interest in social issues, including temperance, prostitution, and suffrage. In her closing remarks she appealed to the nursing profession to share its knowledge and work with suffrage societies in their efforts to improve society.[24] Following Breckinridge's speech, Annie Goodrich spoke to the group and echoed Breckinridge's praise of nursing describing the remarkable strides made in ". . . organization, unity of purpose, strength, professional progress and above all . . . service to render to the race."[25]

At the American Nurses Association's (ANA) fifteenth annual convention held between the 5th and 7th of June, 1912, which overlapped with the Superintendents' eighteenth annual convention, ANA's president, Sarah Sly (1870–1944), was ill and unable to personally deliver her opening speech. In spite of her absence, Sly had her important suffrage-laced address entitled "Our Responsibilities," read to the audience in attendance at the convention. In her address, Sly reviewed the recent progress nursing had made and emphasized the important influence woman suffrage would have on improving the social and health problems confronting society. Sly further advocated health care access for all people saying that, "people must have care."[26] Sly explained that the woman suffrage movement had been underway for more than fifty years and finally, in 1912, had also made progress. President Sly wrote that the franchise would facilitate the changes that women wanted to make in society in order to improve social and economic conditions. She considered suffrage a woman's right as well as a political means to make the world a better place in which to live. Stressing a connection between woman suffrage and nursing, Sly concluded her speech by reiterating the important influence nurses would have if they could vote. As a result of nurses' education and training, nurses could "see those conditions as many others have not the opportunity to see them" and thus, could effectively use the vote to promote desired social change.[27]

Chicago lawyer and former first vice-president of the National American Woman Suffrage Association (1910–1911), Catherine Waugh McCulloch (1862–1945), delivered the opening address at the ANA's fifteenth annual convention. McCulloch spoke directly to the issues surrounding woman's rights and assured nurses that no one could ever accuse them, like other women, of entering male dominated professions and of ". . . taking bread out of men's mouths."[28] Too often women who entered the field of bookkeeping, law, or stenography would experience such accusations. McCulloch continued that government contributed to and sanctioned the belief that perpetuated women's political inferior status, and until women became franchised, they would never by considered politically or economically equal with men. The suffragist speaker invited nurses to join together so that all women:

> *. . . may be free and equal in the eye of the law, so that we may be able to do our work without undue restriction, so that we may be able to protect the helpless and the weak.*[29]

Later during the convention, the ANA membership finally supported the pro-suffrage sentiments expressed by its president, Sarah Sly, and guest speaker Catharine Waugh McCulloch.

NURSES SUPPORT WOMAN SUFFRAGE RESOLUTION

For the first time as a professional group, nurses at the ANA's fifteenth annual convention held between the 5th and the 7th of June, 1912, endorsed an organizational woman suffrage resolution. During one of the discussions leading up to nursing's support of woman suffrage, Annie Goodrich reminded the membership of Lavinia Dock's earlier request to send an international delegation to the ICN prepared to vote on women suffrage. Goodrich asked, "Shall we vote for suffrage or shall we vote against equal suffrage?" She continued by making a motion ". . . that the association put itself on record as in favor of woman suffrage."[30] Sophia Palmer requested the "privilege and honor of seconding the motion."[31] Jane Delano, former international delegate to the ICN held in London, spoke immediately following Palmer's request.

Delano explained that she had always advocated woman suffrage and consequently did not want this year's ICN delegation to be embarrassed by a negative suffrage vote as she had been at the previous convention in London. Sensitive to Lavinia Dock's strong sentiment on the issue, Isabel McIsaac said, "We cannot possibly let it go negatively this time. How in the world will we ever face Miss Dock if we do?"[32]

Delegates from state nursing associations discussed their reasons for supporting this suffrage resolution and the ethics involved with voting for the constituency they represented. One delegate to the ANA convention asked if they had any right to put themselves on record as to what their "personal convictions may be?"[33] Mrs. Colvin, vice-president of the ANA, responded that delegates should be able to speak for their association's membership. Someone else raised the following question: Suppose their personal opinion differed from the state nursing associations they represented? Colvin answered that each delegate had a right to oppose the resolution. However, several delegates said that they already had received their state nursing association's full support to vote for a woman suffrage resolution. Prior to the convention, those delegates had canvassed their constituents on the suffrage issue. One delegate, Davis, told the group that her state association had already voted to support suffrage three years before.

The delegates continued to discuss the necessity for the professional nursing organizations' support of a woman suffrage resolution. Without the vote, many argued, the needed legislative changes promoting the professional practice of nursing and protecting public health stood little chance of passing. State registration of nurses, essential to the profession and to the public, galvanized nursing's support of suffrage. Mary Gladwin (1861–1939), president of the Ohio State Nurses' Association, spoke of the battle among nurses in Ohio over support of suffrage and the relief they would feel if the ANA supported it.

> . . . we had a tremendous fight in Ohio over woman suffrage, and if I go home and tell them that this association approved of woman suffrage it is going to be of very great advantage to us, because state registration in Ohio depends on woman suffrage.[34]

Minnie Ahrens suggested converting nurses into suffrage supporters by appointing them to legislative committees and sending "them down to the capital to try and get along."[35] Clara Noyes (1869–1936), elected president of the National League of Nursing Education (NLNE) in 1913, placed herself on record as endorsing the American Nurses' Association suffrage resolution. Only Adda Eldridge (1864–1955), president of the Illinois State Association for Graduate Nurses (and future president of the ANA) expressed that she had no "definite convictions" about suffrage, and Illinois nurses, whom she represented, had also not committed themselves. Nevertheless, Eldridge felt that because many Illinois nurses strongly advocated woman suffrage it would do less harm to favor the resolution than to do otherwise. Following discussion of the resolution, the ANA took a vote and the "ayes" had it. The American Nurses' Association went on record as supporting woman suffrage.

The July 1912 issue of the *AJN* reported that the overwhelming attendance and the great progress that was made in Chicago had distinguished the 1912 convention as the "greatest ever held."[36] That year, the ANA and the NLNE had met together at their annual conventions in Chicago and as a result important changes occurred in nursing. While at the Chicago meeting, the Superintendents' Society had renamed itself the National League of Nursing Education, public health nurses formed the National Organization for Public Health Nursing (NOPHN), and the American Nurses' Association officially endorsed an organizational woman suffrage resolution. The passage of the woman suffrage resolution was duly noted as "a step forward" for nursing by the *AJN*'s editorial staff in the July issue.[37]

The nursing profession took another step forward in Cologne, Germany, as the Fifth International Congress of Nurses convened and unanimously passed an international woman suffrage resolution. Lavinia Dock's editorial in the September 1912 issue of the *AJN* described the wonderful welcome nurses had received while in Cologne. Women in the host country provided the international group of nurses with several planned receptions, various programs, and free tickets to museums and art shows. Dock reported the results of that congress to the readers and focused on the unity expressed among nurses on the issues of woman suffrage and nurse registration. Votes on each resolution, Dock wrote, had been "adopted unanimously."[38] American nursing that year shared the victory and a growing commitment to woman's rights with the international nursing community. At that Cologne meeting, the international congress voted for American nursing leader Annie Goodrich as its next president and accepted San Francisco's invitation to host the triennial congress in 1915.

American nurses at home read about the successful passage of the woman suffrage and nurse registration resolutions. "Nursing News," featured in September's issue of *AJN* that year, printed the two resolutions for its readers. Passage of both signified the growing tie between the profession and other women's groups. Nursing's high regard for women's efforts to improve world conditions and nursing's need to protect the public from inadequately prepared nurses contributed to the profession's ". . . adherence to the principle of woman suffrage."[39]

Despite the success in Cologne, Lavinia Dock continued to write about women's issues and to convert new suffrage supporters among American nurses. In December 1912, Dock instructed nurses to assess the close relationship between the woman's vote and control of woman's health issues. Dock used as an example an international problem known as "white slavery." She reported on England's proposed passage of "The Criminal Law Amendment Bill" that would prohibit the flagrant practice of international trafficking of women. Dock, however, pointed to the bill's inadequacies, noting that only a special constable rather than an ordinary policemen would be able to arrest a trafficker, making the bill worthless. In light of that deficiency, an "uneasy anti-suffrage member" in the English House of Commons said that women were justified "in demanding the vote on the ground that men do not protect women."[40]

Nursing's international support of woman suffrage in 1912 signified a turning point in history for American nursing, and the woman suffrage movement continued to gain the support of the nursing profession. In 1913, one year after the ANA's endorsement of woman suffrage, the *AJN* reversed its outdated neutral stand towards suffrage to comply with the professional nursing organizations' new policy. American nurses marched in suffrage campaigns and gained greater support for woman suffrage among their profession. Suffragist Lavinia Dock unequivocally linked nursing and women's groups together, saying that the nursing movement was, "a part of the woman movement in its entire program."[41]

Taking part in the woman movement, trained nurses marched together in a suffrage procession held on March 3, 1913, in Washington,

D.C. Nurses had formed a suffrage committee to organize a nursing section for the March parade, and had included nursing leaders Lavinia L. Dock, Estelle L. Wheeler, Isabel McIsaac, Jane A. Delano, Georgia M. Nevins, Reba J. Taylor, and Lily Kanely.[42] The *AJN* published Isabel McIsaac's account of the March 3rd parade and openly supported McIsaac's suffragist sentiments. The journal's editor justified this shift in policy because the journal represented the official policy of the ANA and thus, following the fifteenth annual convention in Chicago in 1912, could now openly endorse woman suffrage.[43]

McIsaac described how a small group of forty or more nurses marched together along Pennsylvania Avenue under the banner of Florence Nightingale. Many more nurses, she said, had marched together with their own state suffrage leagues. Nurses paraded between the section of homemakers and the section of college women. Although they marched orderly at first, pressing forward along the wide avenue, they were interrupted by hecklers as the march progressed. Waiting up to twenty minutes at a time to proceed, many of the participants showed outward signs of courage as they inwardly felt "fear and righteous wrath against those who were responsible for the disorder."[44] Even though the hecklers called out to the nursing section asking, "which of us was Florence," McIsaac felt the nurses received better treatment than the other groups. Perhaps, she said, that they were treated better than others because "even the worst of men" could recall being nursed by one of them.[45]

The marchers appreciated the help troopers on horseback gave to the police who had fumbled control of hecklers all afternoon. Yet this experience opened the eyes of those who marched as to the "depths which will never be closed until women help to do it."[46] In order for women to overcome the kind of hostility and anger expressed by the parade's bystanders, women had to join together toward equal suffrage.

Nurses' support of woman suffrage continued to be reported from different state and alumnae nursing associations in the *AJN*. Members of the Graduate Nurses' Association from the District of Columbia wrote of their support for those marching in the recent suffrage parade described by McIsaac in the April 1913 issue. Although they had not taken any action as a nursing group, eighteen individual nurses had pledged their support for woman suffrage.[47] In the same issue, a brief announcement reported that an "interesting talk on Woman Suffrage" was given at the Hartford Hospital Training School Alumnae Association in Connecticut.[48]

In 1913, at the NLNE's nineteenth annual convention and the ANA's sixteenth annual convention, which met jointly in Atlantic City, New Jersey, Adelaide Nutting, one of the four selected delegates to the International Congress, reported to both groups about her experiences at the previous year's Fifth International Congress of Nurses in Germany. Nutting praised the unified international endorsement of woman suffrage and expressed how pleased she had been to announce the ANA's and the NLNE's support for the resolution at the international meeting.[49]

The host city's Mayor Riddle welcomed the ANA's sixteenth annual convention and opened his address with an anecdote on woman suffrage. Riddle spoke of how his wife had recently become "a suffragette," after hearing an address given by suffragist Dr. Anna Shaw. Following his wife's conversion, Mayor Riddle said, he wrote to Dr. Shaw and pledged support for woman suffrage from himself and his five sons. Acting president of ANA Isabel McIsaac responded to Mayor Riddle's comment, saying that they all were "ardent suffragettes."[50]

At the convention, Lavinia Dock presented an important paper entitled, "Status of the Nurse in the Working World." Dock said that since the audience would hardly expect her to open her mouth "without speaking suffrage," she spoke about the needs of workers for woman suffrage.[51] She proceeded to classify three areas she considered important for all workers: education, shorter hours, and a living wage. However, without the right to vote, none of those areas could be safeguarded or protected by needed legislation. Thus, Dock wrote, "for the sake of the working woman, whose foothold is less secure than ours, no nurse should be opposed to enfranchisement for women."[52] Nurses had a responsibility to assist those in the labor movement because Dock saw it as a "variant" of their own movement.

Nursing suffragists persuaded others to support woman suffrage using control of nursing practice as their primary rationale. Although all women shared similar obstacles to gaining their personal and professional goals without the ballot, nursing faced particularly difficult legislative battles demanding state nurse registration laws, shorter work hours for pupil nurses, and public health reforms.

The following year at the National League of Nursing Education's twentieth annual convention held in 1914, Lavinia Dock's brother, Dr. George Dock, spoke. Like Lavinia, he too was an outspoken advocate of nursing and of woman suffrage. In his paper, presented as part of a series of lectures entitled "The Standardization of Nursing Education," George Dock spoke on the "Essentials of Education," and noted how nursing practice and education had changed through the years to accommodate the increasing complexity of medicine in the early twentieth century. He also acknowledged that nursing, "being one of the fundamental feminine activities," was inextricably associated with the feminist movement. George Dock spoke of the long overdue nurse registration legislation and felt that while no one would argue the efficacy of testing a nurse's competence to practice safely, society moved very slowly to change its laws. He saw no difference in the way society addressed other important social reforms and laws controlling divorce, child labor, pure food, age of consent, woman suffrage, and transportation. These other social issues faced a similar predicament as nurses' registration. Although slow legislation resulted from the outdated notion of states' rights, George Dock informed the group that nursing registration was one reform that could not wait until states' rights were eliminated.[53]

In another paper presented at the twentieth annual convention, where George Dock had just spoken, Adda Eldridge (1864–1955), from St. Luke's Hospital in Chicago, argued the case for woman suffrage in an address entitled, "The Progress of the Past Year in Nursing Legislation and Some Lines of Future Effort." Eldridge spoke during a Saturday morning session on April 25, 1914, at a joint ANA and NLNE meeting. Eldridge presented the results of a survey she had completed using state boards of examiners across the United States as her sample. Eldridge compiled information on the progress of state nurses' registration from the letters she received from state boards. State by state, she described the progress made towards passage of, and in some instances, the improvement of, such legislation. Eldridge included Ohio's letter exactly as it had been sent as she felt "nothing could be omitted or added . . . ."[54] Ohio nurses struggled with the enforcement of a state law which prohibited women from serving on state boards. Because women were not part of the electorate, they were unable to hold state board positions. However, the letter continued, some exceptions to this rule existed since some women were appointed to serve on state boards. Ohio nurses wanted to establish a state board of examiners which would include nurses and introduced this as a new bill before the Ohio legislature in 1913. Although defeated, an amendment to the constitution was passed in November 1913 that allowed women to serve on boards that were involved with issues concerning women or children. Nursing leaders used this new amendment to convince Ohio legislators that nurses should be allowed to serve on the state boards which regulated the licensure exams for nurse registration. Legislators consequently reworded a new bill requesting that the state medical board "employ five nurses to examine nurses."[55] In spite of their efforts, the state attorney general ruled that the exception to women serving on boards did not apply to nurse boards of examiners. He erroneously reasoned that the nursing board did not involve the "interests and care of women or children or both."[56] Nurses then urged the governor of Ohio to support their bill and send it to a special legislative session in January 1914. The governor denied their request, thereby making Ohio nurses realize how desperately they needed woman suffrage to make legislative changes.[57]

Eldridge described how West Virginia nurses faced a dilemma similar to those in Ohio, and they too advocated woman suffrage as a result. In 1907, West Virginia had passed a state nurse registration law that notably improved professional standards. However, nurses excluded from board membership wanted these political appointments and recognized that woman suffrage was needed in order "to place nurses on board."[58]

Eldridge urged nurses to collectively educate the public as to the importance of nurse registration. She believed that society needed to be informed on how such legislation would protect them from underprepared and poorly trained nurses and emphatically said, "Publicity and Education! Make the public demand laws to protect themselves."[59] Nursing wanted the American public to be a political ally as nurses politically lobbied for a controlling voice in their profession.

Following Eldridge's speech at the twentieth annual NLNE convention, Lila Pickhardt from the Pasadena Hospital Association, Pasadena, California, spoke on "Recent Legislation Governing Hours of Duty of Pupil Nurses in Hospitals." Pickhardt presented a history of women labor laws as background for her argument to shorten pupil nurse work hours from twelve hours and longer to an eight-hour work day. She explained that only in those states where women could vote did an eight-hour work day law exist. Long hours of overwork caused fatigue and health problems among women and these same arguments could be raised in regards to the "superhuman endurance" demanded of pupil nurses by unsympathetic hospital boards. While California's eight-hour law benefitted nursing students, governmental control of nursing hours was highly controversial for both hospitals and nurses.[60]

The ANA and the NLNE met jointly at many of their national conventions but did not include the National Association of Colored Graduate Nurses (NACGN) in their proceedings. Although the NACGN convention minutes do not reveal any direct endorsement of a resolution for woman suffrage, the NACGN maintained a relationship with the International Council of Nurses (ICN), which did. Members at the NACGN's seventh annual convention again voted to send a representative to the International Council to be convened in California in 1915. Believing that such participation was important, the NACGN further supported the elected candidate, identified in the minutes as C. Morgan, by defraying the delegate's cost to the meeting. However, a Miss Sharp, noted as a delegate to the International Congress, stated that she could not present a report at the NACGN's eighth annual convention because the congress had not met because of the European War.[61]

While war raged in Europe and prevented many of the ICN's European members from attending the 1915 international nursing convention, the ANA and the NLNE held their respective 1915 conventions in San Francisco as originally planned. By 1915, the woman suffrage movement had gained increasing attention and support from nursing organizations that openly endorsed the congressional passage of the Susan B. Anthony bill. The ANA, the NLNE, and the newly formed National Organization for Public Health Nursing (NOPHN) officially cast their joint support for the Susan B. Anthony amendment.

At the NLNE's twenty-first annual convention held in June 1915, President Clara Noyes opened a joint session of the ANA, the NLNE, and the NOPHN asking nurses to unify and protect the profession and the public from "charlatanism and quackery."[62] Noyes felt that at no other time in nursing's history had the demand for the "highly educated and carefully prepared women" been as great as it was in 1915. Noyes called for a uniformity in use of the term "nurse" and in the entrance requirements for nurses. She also wanted nurses to unite their efforts in order to campaign for financial endowments for nursing schools, improve educational standards, and actively support their state nurse registration campaign. Knowing the barriers nursing would face in its efforts to enact these professional reforms, Noyes encouraged the audience to learn from other movements in America's history which required unified strength and fortitude. She cited as examples those social movements that emancipated the slaves and obtained freedom of the press and free education.[63]

Throughout the 1915 annual convention of both the ANA and the NLNE, increasing references to woman suffrage and the larger woman movement appeared.[64] Following the delivery of Noyes's presidential address, Sara Parsons (1864–1949) presented the publicity committee's report. Parsons explained that since the NLNE's publicity committee hoped to attract the "best womanhood in our country" into the nursing profession, the committee urged nursing organizations to affiliate with other women's clubs and show "a helpful spirit towards all activities for the public welfare."[65] By doing so, Parsons believed that nursing would gain greater public respect and become a more attractive career prospect for women. During the discussion following the publicity committee's report, Parsons suggested that each state nursing association hire a public spokesperson who would speak on its behalf at women's clubs throughout the country. She believed that women and nursing had a great deal to gain from each other's support, especially in states where women voted. Parsons concluded by saying:

> *If the women of the country, especially in those states where we have suffrage, should rise up and demand that our nurses' schools should be what they ought to be and that nurses should have a legal status, I think there would be something great accomplished.*[66]

During the 1915 NLNE convention, president Clara Noyes again addressed the group and introduced the topic of suffrage by reminding the audience of the ANA's 1912 unanimous decision to support the woman suffrage resolution. Although Noyes assured the NLNE members that their twenty-first convention was not a suffrage meeting, nevertheless, they had the opportunity to hear Miss Whitney from the

Congressional Union (CU) speak on congressional efforts for suffrage.[67] Whitney informed nurses of the two political methods by which to pass woman suffrage. The first method, initially supported by the CU, encouraged each state to support woman suffrage. However, the CU changed its approach when it became abundantly clear that such a method proved to be too "slow and inefficient."[68] Although Wyoming had been the first state to grant woman suffrage in 1869, by 1915 only eleven states had followed its example. The second strategy used by the CU to obtain woman suffrage sought the passage of a federal amendment to the Constitution. Whitney urged nurses to professionally and personally support the federal woman suffrage amendment known as the Susan B. Anthony Amendment and proceeded to read to the nursing audience the following resolution:

> *The right of the citizens of the United States to vote shall not be denied * * * or abridged by the United States or by any state because of sex.*[69]

In accordance with the speaker's request, the members at the meeting proposed a resolution to support the Susan B. Anthony Amendment. Annie Goodrich endorsed it and the NLNE passed the following resolution:

> *WHEREAS the enfranchisement of women, the recognition of the political rights of one-half the people of the United States to have a voice in the decision of questions of vital interest to them, such as peace and war, child labor, marriage and divorce, community of property, etc., is the foremost political issue of the day,*
>
> Therefore be it resolved *that the National League of Nursing Education in convention assembled in San Francisco, June 24, 1915, endorse the Susan B. Anthony Amendment, known in the 63rd Congress as the Bristow-Mendell Amendment, and urge its passage by the 64th Congress.*[70]

The interest in suffrage echoed at the ANA's eighteenth annual convention taking place that same week in San Francisco. At the Friday morning session held on June 25, 1915, at the ANA convention, woman's rights appeared on the agenda. The first discussion that morning related to an address given by a representative from the National Council of Trained Nurses of Great Britain and Ireland, a Miss Kent, who attended the ANA convention. Miss Kent had planned to attend the previously scheduled International Council of Nurses meeting (ICN); however, because of the European war the international congress was suspended. In spite of the drain the war placed on European nurses, Miss Kent came to San Francisco to attend the ANA convention. In Kent's address, she spoke of the sadness her delegation felt leaving their own "bleeding country" and of the "abundant kindness and hospitality" they received in America. She greatly admired American nursing for the solidarity it displayed, the work of the organizations, and the excellent *AJN*. More pointedly, Kent admired the forwardness American nursing displayed in the political arena. She said, "You have political enfranchisement and you have professional enfranchisement."[71]

In addition to the British delegation, other foreign delegations made their way to the convention despite of war. Annie Goodrich acknowledged their presence at the meeting, welcoming representatives from Holland, Canada, New Zealand, India, and Australia. Goodrich said that even as the world experiences the "terrible sorrow" of war, nurses meet as an international unified body. Like a family, all shared in the impoverishment war rendered to all mankind. Goodrich spoke of future international nursing meetings to be held following the war when delegations would come together to overcome the poverty and distress war would bring. Visionary in her comments, she believed that within the twentieth century we would see the "death warrant of war" signed. Goodrich described a united international nursing community to lead the world in its efforts for peace, expressing her belief that ". . . nurses could really talk intelligently and consistently about the brotherhood of man."[72]

The second item at the June 25 meeting was a resolution which appealed to Harvard University to "admit women to the Public Health Course" who were qualified but were denied admissions because of gender. This motion carried, thus indicating professional nursing's concern for opportunities denied them based on sexist criteria.[73]

The third item broached that morning reflected the suffrage mood that had been evident the day before at the NLNE convention. Effie J. Taylor read a motion similar to the one already passed the previous day at the NLNE meeting endorsing the Susan B. Anthony Amendment. A Miss Sweeney moved that the ANA adopt the suffrage motion, a Miss Peterson seconded it, and the ANA voted to officially endorse woman suffrage.[74]

Immediately following the ANA's endorsement of the Susan B. Anthony Amendment, the director of the Bureau of the Registration of

Nurses in California and leader in the California State Nurses' Association, Anna Jammé (1867–1939), reminded the ANA of its earlier 1908 defeat of a woman suffrage resolution while in San Francisco. Jammé spoke of how Lavinia Dock at that time was "so bitterly disappointed" that Dock never fully recovered. Thus, Jammé recommended that the ANA send a telegram to Dock informing her of the association's new position on woman suffrage, believing that this would be a "courteous and humane act." In accordance with Jammé's request, the members of the ANA unanimously approved and widely applauded her thoughtful suggestion.[75]

Lavinia Dock's absence was felt at the 1915 convention and had been noticed by Annie Goodrich, president of the International Council of Nurses. Goodrich voiced her disappointment at missing Dock when she gave the ICN's report instead of Dock, the INC's secretary. Goodrich told how Dock was a woman of "concentrated" interests and intensely involved with woman suffrage; therefore, as a result of such passion, Dock had stayed in New York City to press for woman's rights instead of attending the San Francisco convention. In full support of her colleague, Goodrich said, "I am sure the work she is rendering for the nurse in obtaining the vote for women in New York City will quite repay us for her absence from this congress . . . ."[76]

The momentous decisions of the 1915 convention held in San Francisco echoed the feelings of many nurses in the professional community and were accordingly expressed in their professional journal. America's nursing community unanimously supported woman suffrage, wrote D. Elva Mills Stanley, R.N., in her article, "Nursing and Citizenship," which appeared in the October 1915 issue of the *AJN*. One year prior to Stanley's article, she had presented this same paper before the Indiana Federation of Women's Clubs in Evansville, Indiana. To Stanley, the ANA, the NLNE, and the NOPHN's collective support of woman suffrage would ultimately improve the health of Americans. She described how nurses and the Indiana's women's club could join forces "to strengthen our arm and hasten the fulfillment of our desires." Nurses who worked in hospitals, schools, homes, and factories could use those opportunities to teach their patients and families in the community about health, hygiene, and sanitation. In many instances, members of the women's club already worked with nurses in those areas and already saw the value of trained nurses in promoting healthy behaviors. Stanley asked for cooperation in demanding state laws protecting the licensure of trained nurses which assured the public better qualified nurses and thus better health care for the public.[77]

Throughout the country, trained nurses responded favorably to the increased efforts of the woman's movement and in some instances openly affiliated with other women's groups. In 1915, the Mississippi State Association of Graduate Nurses (MSAGN) joined the Mississippi State Federation of Women's Clubs when asked to do so by the women's club. The MSAGN and the women's federation both recognized that working together promoted the interests of their respective organizations. In 1915, the MSAGN, organized only three years before and with sixty-five members, had successfully passed a state registration act which the Mississippi governor signed on March 11, 1914. Following the signing of the bill, the MSAGN reportedly turned its energies toward outside political issues affecting nursing, women, and health. Thus, when invited, Mississippi nurses joined the Mississippi State Federation of Women's Clubs. Within two years the MSAGN's delegate to the women's federation, along with the other members of the federation, endorsed a resolution supporting woman suffrage.78

At the twenty-second annual convention of the NLNE held in New Orleans, Louisiana, between April 27th and May 3rd, 1916, a call for unity among nurses and women's groups was again expressed by President Clara Noyes. In Noyes's opening address she encouraged the NLNE, the ANA, and the NOPHN to work together in the preparation of "properly prepared and educated women." Without solidarity among trained nurses, they had little hope at ever getting "good nursing laws, proper recognition or good schools of nursing." For success in those areas, nurses needed to stand "shoulder to shoulder and work for them." Noyes referred the audience to an argument she had often heard in regard to women obtaining the suffrage, that "when women really want suffrage, they will get it." For nurses and nurse registration, she said, it was the same thing: "when nurses really want good nursing laws, they will get them." Nurses, like the suffragists, had to unite to bring about political and professional changes.[79]

Reports from various state leagues at the twenty-second convention validated the timely theme expressed by Noyes encouraging nursing to develop ties with other women's groups. At the NLNE twenty-second annual convention, the Michigan State League reported that the Wayne County Equal Suffrage League had sponsored a publicity campaign for nursing. The report given by one Michigan nurse, a Miss Foy, explained that the Equal Suffrage League published a featured article promoting nurses in a paper called, "The Michigan Woman." Although no further discussion was found in the proceedings as to the relationship between the Michigan League for Nurses and the Equal Suffrage League, both groups had worked together on a project that promoted nursing and woman suffrage.[80]

As nursing's ties with outside women's groups became increasingly prevalent, American nurses became more concerned about the war in Europe. America did not enter the war until April 1917, confronting nursing with numerous responsibilities and opportunities to serve its country. In response to these responsibilities and opportunities, professional nursing organizations supplies the American war effort with trained nurses. Attention to the proper qualifications and training of nurses in the military dominated the interest of nursing organizations along with supplying needed nursing care in civilian hospitals and public health. As a result of the war, the United States experienced shortages of properly trained nurses to fill the multiple nursing jobs available in both civilian and military capacities. To accommodate this emergency, nursing educators opened shortened nurse training courses such as the Vassar Training Camp for Nurses at some colleges to prepare college women as qualified nurses.[81]

While war raged in Europe, Dock kept American nurses appraised of the political advances made by women and looked optimistically at Canada as a shining example of social change. At the twenty-third NLNE annual convention held in Philadelphia, while serving as secretary of the International Council of Nurses, Dock praised Canadian nurses for their efforts to improve the status of professional nursing in Canada and also praised them for having successfully achieved "political equality." Dock acknowledged while in the midst of world war, Canadian women from Ontario to the Pacific Ocean became enfranchised citizens of Canada in March 1917. Optimistically she expressed her views "that the outlook for women and their professional progress is wholly bright."[82]

Another paper presented at the same convention where Dock spoke, called for professional progress and social change. The responsibility of American nurses for the social welfare of the community, especially to the civilian community during the war, remained the central theme for

Marie Lockwood, Superintendent of the Visiting Nurse Society of Wilmington, Delaware. In Lockwood's paper entitled, "The Relation of the Private Duty Nurse as a Social Worker," she argued that private-duty nurses had always included social work as part of their nursing role. Lockwood felt this was an important aspect of the nurses' work and one which required additional education to fulfill. Lockwood placed the responsibility of social change on nursing, requiring nurses to affiliate with women's groups so they could accomplish this. She encouraged nurses to "identify themselves with other women's activities and interests" and to avoid settling down in "too narrow a rut." Since women needed an education, economic independence, suffrage, social equality, and friendship in order to "do their duty to themselves and to other neighbors, then how can *nurses* afford to be negative anywhere?"[83] Lockwood concluded by encouraging nurses to improve their education so they might be better prepared to handle the pressing social needs of patients, families, and communities.

Lockwood's paper presented at the twenty-third annual conference of the NLNE reaffirmed the professional progress Dock had described at the same meeting. Additional evidence of the social progress Dock advocated also appeared in the December 1917 issue of the *AJN,* which paid tribute to pioneer suffragist Susan B. Anthony. The *AJN* announced that it had moved its publication office to Rochester, New York, which had been the home of Susan B. Anthony. The journal honored Anthony by carrying a full-page photograph of her on the first page. The editors said the Anthony's portrait served to commemorate "the wonderful suffrage victory which has come to the women of New York State." The voters of New York state, after witnessing an intensive suffrage campaign, had finally passed woman suffrage in their state.[84] The *AJN* editors attributed New York's successful passage of woman suffrage to Anthony's vision and drive and credited her for changing the legal and social status of all women, even in states without suffrage. Finally, the editorial explained that Anthony had known the *AJN* in its early days of publication and had shown personal interest in nursing's struggle for legal recognition, hence clarifying for the nursing readership the close ties that nursing and the woman's movement had previously shared.[85]

In 1918, the professional nursing organizations' support of woman suffrage continued to be strengthened by new suffrage resolutions passed and by affiliations with women's groups interested in social reform. Nurses openly expressed their support for woman suffrage as evidenced in a telegram sent to President Woodrow Wilson. Nurses broadened their professional and personal vision by affiliating with women's organizations and responding to social, political, and economic changes in 1918, thus lifting the narrow blinders believed necessary during the earlier stage of nursing's professional development. Beginning in 1917, suffragists from the Woman's Party campaigned outside of the White House demanding that President Wilson include the woman suffrage amendment on the congressional agenda. Suffragists stood with banners asking Wilson for the same democratic rights for women at home as the country fought to defend the democratic rights of others in Europe. The banners held silently by women activists represented the "weapons of war" and simply asked the questions: "Mr. President, What Will You Do For Woman Suffrage," and "How Long Must Women Wait for Liberty." Women in their many different organizations sent telegrams to the president protesting the passage of wartime legislation without women's consent. In spite of the peaceful nature of their inquiry, the government responded to the suffragists' picketing and marches with arrests and imprisonments. Nursing's suffragist, Lavinia Dock, was among one of the first groups of picketing activists that faced the government's suppression and was jailed for three days in June of 1917 and again in November 1917 for fifteen days.[86]

Like so many other American organizations, nursing's professional associations sent telegrams protesting the lack of woman suffrage in America to President Wilson. On May 11, 1918, the executive board of the NLNE voted to publicly endorse the federal suffrage amendment and expressed this support in a telegram sent to the president of the United States. At that meeting the board passed the following resolution:

> *It was moved by Miss Powell and seconded by Miss Jammé that a resolution favoring the federal suffrage amendment be sent to Congress.*[87]

Suffragist organizations reaffirmed their commitment to woman suffrage even as the national war effort demanded that women use their time for other, war-related activities. Professional nursing organizations also experienced the increased demands war placed on the supply of nurses in Europe and at home. Nevertheless, nursing reaffirmed its commitment to professional goals. Throughout 1918, the

NLNE continued to maintain high educational standards for nurse training while attempting to meet their patriotic duty. While campaigning to attract new recruits into schools of nursing, members of the NLNE spoke at women's groups, clubs, and schools in the hope of finding newcomers to the profession. The various reports of state leagues and speeches heard in the proceedings of the joint meeting of the NLN, the ANA, and the NOPHN held in May 1918 in Cleveland, Ohio, bear witness to this alliance.

At a joint meeting of three national nursing organizations representing more than 40,000 graduate nurses, the opening addresses reflected the patriotic concerns of nursing during World War I. At the May meeting in 1918 the presidents were Lillian Clayton of the NLNE, Mary Beard of the NOPHN, and Annie Goodrich of the American Nurses' Association. Each president offered nursing service to the country at this time of national crisis. Whether nursing the community or nursing the troops, their work was considered central to America's success in world events. Annie Goodrich reiterated a common theme for unity among sister organizations; however, in 1918, the call for unity related to nurses' ability to better serve the country's needs during the war. She stated that "ours is essentially a woman's problem" and cooperation of the women's organizations was central to the solutions.[88]

In her opening address at the twenty-fourth annual convention of the NLNE, president S. Lillian Clayton said that the nursing organization would meet the world's need for qualified nurses because it was its "responsibility to do so."[89] While the NLNE attempted to find enough qualified nurses to meet the national need for nurses, the leaders of the NLNE also tried to meet the nurses' professional need for recognition for the nursing services they rendered. In the military, specifically the Army Nurse Corps, rank for nurses would have brought the desired acknowledgment and recognition that trained nurses wanted and deserved. Since nurses did not have relative rank with men in the military serving in similar posts, reducing this inequality became a heated debate among the members of nursing organizations. Without rank, a nurse's authority in making decisions while caring for the sick and wounded remained challenged and threatened. Many nurses wrote home from the World War I battlefields of the "thorny path" they faced when challenged by ". . . men who never have been brought up to respect women's orders."[90] Nurses in May 1918 supported a resolution brought before the congress by a "group of lay women" endorsing a federal bill for the ranking of trained graduate nurses in the army and the navy. This was passed at the May 11, 1918, joint session of the ANA, the NLNE, and the NOPHN held in Ohio.[91]

While many nurses supported America's war effort, some nursing leaders supported the woman's peace movement. Nursing settlement house leader Lillian Wald opposed the war and had joined the Woman's Peace Party along with other prominent women in the reform movement such as Chicago's Jane Addams. Two years before America entered the war, in 1915, American nurses had read of the activities of the Woman's Peace Party in Lavinia Dock's featured "Foreign Department" column in the *AJN*. Dock had published the Woman's Peace Party proclamation that women no longer had to consent to war's "reckless destruction."[92] In addition to opposing war, women claimed the right to partake in the decisions of government leading up to war. They demanded that women share in "deciding between war and peace in all the courts of high debate; within the home, the school, . . . and the State."[93] Thus, Dock clearly illustrated that in wanting peace, women wanted suffrage.

Woman suffrage also appeared on the agenda of the same 1918 joint annual conventions of the NLNE, the ANA, and the NOPHN. Nursing representatives of the three organizations sent another telegram from nursing to President Wilson urging him to persuade Congress to pass the federal amendment on woman suffrage:

> . . . *by bringing the members of the National Legislature to a realization that a democracy cannot consistently discriminat* [sic] *between the man and woman citizen, and asking him to see that the right to vote be granted to women.*[94]

The 1918 joint national conventions held by the three professional nursing organizations reaffirmed nurses' political support of woman suffrage. A coalition among women's groups and nursing emerged as state nursing associations sought to learn more about women's issues and to gather support for nursing issues such as nurse recruitment, better nursing education, and state nursing registration. At the NLNE's twenty-fourth annual convention, the Ohio State League of Nursing Education reported growing interest in woman suffrage and considered it one of the most socially and politically relevant topics discussed at monthly Ohio State League meetings.[95] At the same meeting, nurses in South Carolina described their struggle to serve on state boards because their state constitution still prohibited women from holding political office. As a result of this outdated political prohibition, the South Carolina state nursing association had to vigorously lobby its state legislators to be represented on the state board of directors that controlled the licensing of nurses. The composition of the board of directors, consisting solely of male physicians, changed to include six women after extensive campaigning by nurses. However, the South Carolina nurses reported that the women could attend board sessions, but could not grade the practical examinations for nursing licensure.[96]

The affiliation with women in clubs throughout the country served the interests of the professional nursing associations both at the state and the national level. The South Carolina state nurses association reported at the Ohio meeting that it had established a close relationship with the strong body of Federated Women's Clubs of South Carolina and that the Federated Women's Clubs had assisted the association in publicizing the activities of the state nurses association. On the national level, the secretary of the ANA in 1918, Katherine DeWitt (1867–1963), reported in the twenty-first annual proceedings that the ANA had recently joined the General Federation of Women's Clubs.[97]

In 1919, the final year of the suffrage campaign led by women's rights activists, nursing congratulated Illinois for ratifying the federal suffrage amendment, again telegrammed their support for woman suffrage to the president of the United States, and argued for woman suffrage as the only way to obtain military rank for nurses. Additionally that year, African-American nurses were called on to support woman suffrage by Adah Thoms, the president of the National Association of Colored Graduate Nurses.

At the twenty-fifth annual NLNE convention held in Chicago in June 1919, [Mrs.] Ira Couch Wood, the director of the Elizabeth McCormick Memorial Fund in Chicago, joyously referred to the Illinois ratification of the federal suffrage amendment and happily proclaimed:

> *Last night we had a suffrage jubilee here in Illinois, rejoicing over the fact that Illinois was the very first state to ratify the suffrage amendment. I am perfectly sure that in all the states you are going to follow and ratify the amendment in a very short time, and then freedom of women for all ages is going to be a reality in a very, very short time.[98]*

Wood continued by saying that although American women were among the last in the world to earn the right to vote, she hoped they would be first to take advantage of it. Consequently, women needed an opportunity to become educated and prepare themselves for political citizenship. Wood warned her audience that woman suffrage would be useless if women were prohibited from equal educational opportunities or were barred from becoming political leaders. In addition to Wood's plea for equal educational opportunities, she stressed the importance of finding financial endowments for women's education equivalent to those found in men's schools. The need for better education to prepare women to become better citizens struck a familiar chord with nursing organizations that similarly struggled to maintain their educational standards in order to graduate better prepared nurses. While the country demanded shorter nurse training to accommodate nursing shortages which resulted from the war and from the deadly flu epidemic of 1918–1919, nursing leaders in the professional organizations held fast to their belief that better educated nurses, like better educated women, would make them better citizens. Wood warned the NLNE that nursing would never achieve "the real recognition . . . as one of the greatest professions for women," unless the public financially endowed nursing and nursing education "with the same generosity that they make for men for all forms of education."[99]

While American nurses fought the battle of war in European hospitals and struggled with the overwhelmingly high death rate of the influenza epidemic at home, publication of the proceedings of the 1918 twenty-fourth annual report of the NLNE was delayed one year. Because of the war and the outbreak of the epidemic, it was too difficult to find a publisher and nurses had to wait a year before they could read that the NLNE executive board had supported the federal suffrage amendment. In the published proceedings, NLNE secretary Laura Logan wrote in her report that "it was voted that a resolution favoring the Federal Suffrage Amendment should be sent to Congress."[100]

Although the war delayed the publication of the NLNE proceedings, it accelerated the argument of rank for nurses and the need for woman suffrage to successfully obtain rank. Helen Hoy Greeley, during a discussion on military rank for nurses at the twenty-fifth NLNE annual convention in 1919, argued that rank for nurses in the military was just one of the programs that womanhood, not just nurses, should adopt as a result of the war. Anna Maxwell (1851–1929) further contended that to acquire military rank for nurses required unity among all nurses. In the same discussion, former president of the NLNE, Clara Noyes, asserted that although some women did not want equal rank for nurses in the military, that was not a sufficient reason to oppose military rank anymore than those who did not want woman suffrage gave sufficient reason to oppose suffrage. Military rank, like equal suffrage, was "just one step onward."[101]

The plea for unity among nurses of the NLNE, the ANA, and the NOPHN did not extend to include the African-American nurses who were members of the National Association of Colored Graduate Nurses. Omitted from joint decisions of the NLNE, the ANA, and the NOPHN, the black nursing association faced isolation from unified suffrage resolutions and from unified arguments favoring military rank for nurses. Nevertheless, the president of the National Association of Colored Graduates, Adah Thoms, in her opening address at the twelfth annual convention held in Boston, Massachusetts, in August 1919, petitioned African-American nurses to exercise the ballot wherever they could vote. Thoms urged nurses "to take advantage of the scholarships that the surgeon general offers . . . and to use the ballots in the states where women are franchised."[102]

In the spring of 1920, as women suffragists were close to successfully passing the federal suffrage amendment and thus gaining control of their political lives, trained nurses continued the struggle to control their own profession. The events of the twenty-sixth annual meeting of the NLNE held in Atlanta, Georgia, in April 1920 reflected this professional conflict. During a discussion at the 1920 meeting, the NLNE membership entertained the idea of a bylaw change which would open voting privileges to lay members. Some NLNE members questioned the efficacy of such an idea and were concerned that if physicians were allowed voting privileges they might try to exert medical control over nursing education and practice. NLNE secretary Laura Logan (1879–1974) raised the issue that physicians perceived nurses as handmaidens rather than as public servants, and that physicians had no use for nursing education. Thus, Logan felt that nurses had to "protect" their "standards of nursing education until such time as the physician is as broad [minded] as some of the nurses are today." Nursing leaders wanted to move nursing education out of the hospital setting and into colleges and universities. However, nursing educators received no support from medical schools already situated in colleges and universities because, according to Logan, medicine wanted no connection to this kind of progress in nursing education even though medical education had "risen on the shoulders of nursing."[103]

At the Atlanta meeting, NLNE President Anna Jammé responded to the question of lay membership by relaying an experience in California. Jammé referred to a national women's club named the Civic Center. She described the Civic Center as a politically active club that advocated woman suffrage and other protective legislation for women in California. The Civic Center also concerned itself with the nursing shortage which existed at that time and with standards of nursing education. Nevertheless, as concerned as the Civic Center appeared to be, its members were unfamiliar with the work of the National League of Nursing Education. Although the work of the league was familiar to nursing, most of the public knew little about its work because the league had not made itself known to the public: the public "hardly know we exist." Jammé supported a voting lay membership because she believed that such a group could help educate and inform the general public of the work of the National League of Nursing Education. Jammé appreciated the efforts of other women's groups and recognized the benefits that such a coalition could produce for nursing and for women.[104]

Two final speeches presented at the twenty-sixth annual meeting in 1920 applauded nursing's transition into a strong and viable profession for women in the twentieth century. On Friday evening, April 16, 1920, speaker W. P. Morril explained how nursing had advanced from the simple art of bedmaking to much more. "Woman suffrage and prohibition we have attained, prophylaxis we are concentrating on and peace may come, when we have educated the rest of the world . . . ."[105]

Following Morril's speech, nursing educator Adelaide Nutting addressed the convention, and she too reflected on the changes in nursing and in the world during the first twenty years of the twentieth century. Nutting spoke of the progressive reforms in America and how these reforms had influenced nursing's professional growth. Nutting described the changing world in which the nursing profession had first germinated, grown, and matured. She highlighted nursing's reaction to the social, economic, and political reform movements during that period, specifically identifying woman suffrage and prohibition as two reforms which nursing influenced and was itself influenced. Nutting said:

We must, it appears, always and inevitably be affected by any widely pervading social attitude or movement, and we in our turn must in some similar measure affect them. Prohibition and woman suffrage are two of the recent great social movements which will profoundly affect the future of nursing.

Nutting further observed that those progressive reformers in "various branches of industry," who struggled to obtain an eight-hour day, had undoubtedly strengthened nursing's attempts "to secure shorter hours for both student and graduate nurses." Similarly, Nutting saw the influence nursing would have on women's education and said, "our requirements for admission to schools of nursing must have distinct effect upon the education of young women throughout the country (and indeed eventually throughout other countries)."[106] Nutting recognized the contribution that nursing had made and would continue to make in the important social movements of the world. When American women finally earned the franchise in the summer of 1920, nursing had changed from a young profession centered on its own development to a maturing profession ready to respond to world events. Like all women in support of suffrage, nurses recognized the significance of winning a political voice of their own. However, for nursing, the vote meant more than personal equality: the vote represented the avenue for professional advancement and autonomy as well.

On August 26, 1920, 26 million American women of voting age found themselves franchised. During the summer of 1920, the federal suffrage amendment had been ratified and signed into law, giving women from all different backgrounds the opportunity to actively participate in the governing of America. American nursing organizations had contributed to the successful passage of woman suffrage and now faced the challenges of using their political vote.[107]

NOTES

1. Catherine Waugh McCullough [sic], Opening Address during the Proceedings of the Fifteenth Annual Convention of the ANA. *AJN*, 12 no.

11 (August 1912): 866; Paul S. Boyer, Catherine Gouger Waugh Mc-Culloch, in James, James, and Boyer, *Notable American Women,* II:459–60. Catherine Waugh McCulloch was a lawyer in Chicago and a noted speaker on woman suffrage; a discrepancy in the spelling of her last name between the *AJN* (McCullough) and Notable American Women (McCulloch) noted.

2. Flexner, *Century of Struggle: The Woman's Rights Movement,* 256–285. Lavinia Dock, Florence Kelly, Charlotte Perkins Gilman, and Leonora O'Reilly were active in the Equality League of Self-Supporting Women (reorganized as the Women's Political Union), which began in 1907.

3. For discussion of Dock's withdrawal, see Adelaide Nutting, *Proceedings of the Seventeenth Annual Report Convention of the ASSTSN* (Baltimore: J. H. Furst, 1911), 160–161.

4. Editorial Comment, "Suggestions to Organization Workers," *AJN,* 12 no. 1 (October 1911): 5.

5. Mary Johnston, "Editor's Miscellany: The Reason Why," *AJN,* 12 no. 1 (October 1911): 76–77.

6. Lavinia Dock, "Foreign Department," *AJN,* 11 no. 12 (September 1911): 1040.

7. Lavinia Dock, "Foreign Department," *AJN,* 12 no. 2 (November 1911): 129.

8. Ibid.

9. Nursing News and Announcements, "Washington," *AJN,* 11 no. 5 (February 1911): 404; Harper, History of Woman Suffrage, 675. Full suffrage for women in the state of Washington was passed in February of 1909.

10. Nursing News and Announcements, "Maryland," *AJN,* 11 no. 6 (March 1911): 482.

11. "Nursing News and Announcements, Virginia: The Eleventh Meeting of the Graduate Nurses' Association of Virginia," *AJN,* 11 no. 6 (March 1911): 484–485; James, James, and Boyer, Lila Hardaway Meade, *Notable American Women,* 504–505; B. B. Valentine was Lila Hardaway Meade Valentine and married to Benjamin Bathchelder Valentine, whose name was abbreviated in *Nursing News* as B. B. Valentine.

12. Edna Foley, "Department of Visiting Nursing and Social Welfare," *AJN,* 11 no. 7 (April 1911): 554.

13. Lavinia L. Dock, "Nursing News and Announcements: International," *AJN,* 12 no. 1 (October 1911): 58.

14. "Nursing News and Announcements: Indiana," *AJN*, 12 no. 2 (November 1911): 155.

15. Letter from Dock to the NACGN and read by Mrs. Watkins in 1911 at the fourth annual convention of the NACGN, Unpublished proceedings, NACGNR, Schomburg, Box 1, Volume 1, p. 37. Direct support, discussion, or official vote on woman suffrage was not found in the proceedings of the NACGN between 1908 and 1920. However, the connection to the ICN and its international decisions regarding suffrage suggests that the NACGN was knowledgeable about and supportive of the issue.

16. Report of the International Congress in Cologne, Germany, by Rosa Williams at the sixth annual convention of the NACGN, September 3, 1913, Unpublished proceedings, NACGNR, Schomburg, Box 1, Volume 1, pp. 57–58.

17. "Book Reviews: Women in Public Affairs," *AJN*, 13 no. 5 (February 1913): 495. This review was excerpted from "The Progress of the World," in the *American Review of Reviews* for January 1913 and referred to the Progressive Party's work in woman suffrage.

18. "Nursing News and Announcements: Pennsylvania, The Philadelphia General Hospital Alumnae Association," *AJN*, 12 no. 6 (March 1912): 515; see Harper, *History of Woman Suffrage*, 550–64, for a history of woman suffrage in Pennsylvania. The speaker, Mrs. Rudolph Blankenberg, was identified in the *AJN* announcement by her married name, but most likely she was Lucretia Blankenberg of Philadelphia, the president of the State Woman Suffrage Association in Pennsylvania. The Equal Franchise Society was formed in 1909 as an auxiliary of the state association and its membership represented prominent Philadelphian women.

19. Lavinia L. Dock, "Foreign Department: The Cologne Congress," *AJN*, 12 no. 7 (April 1912): 574–5.

20. "Nursing News and Announcements: Virginia, The Graduate Nurses' Association of Virginia," *AJN*, 12 no. 8 (May 1912): 687.

21. "Nursing News," ibid.; see Husted, The *History of Woman Suffrage*, 665–72, for a history of woman suffrage in Virginia. Lila Meade Valentine was the president for eleven years of the Equal Suffrage League of Virginia formed in 1909.

22. "Nursing News and Announcements: Indiana," *AJN*, 12 no. 9 (May 1912): 756.

23. Lavinia L. Dock, "Foreign Department: The Cologne Congress," *AJN*, 12 no. 8 (May 1912): 656.

24. Sophonisba Preston Breckinridge. *Proceedings of the Eighteenth Annual Convention of the ASSTSN* (Springfield, MA: Thatcher Art Printery, 1912), 40–42; Christopher Lasch, Sophonisba Preston Breckinridge, in James, James, and Boyer, *Notable American Women,* I: 233–236.

25. Annie Goodrich, "A General Presentation of the Statutory Requirements of the Different States," *Proceedings of the Eighteenth Annual Convention of the ASSTSN,* 212.

26. Sara E. Sly, "Address of the President: Our Responsibilities: Report of the Fifteenth Annual Convention of the American Nurses' Association," *AJN,* 12 no. 11 (July 1912): 892.

27. Ibid., 893.

28. Catharine Waugh McCulloch, "Proceedings of the Fifteenth Annual Convention of the ANA," 864.

29. Ibid., 868.

30. Annie Goodrich, "Proceedings of the Fifteenth Annual Convention of the ANA," *AJN,* 12 no. 11 (August 1912): 973.

31. Sophia Palmer, "Proceedings of the Fifteenth Annual Convention of the ANA," 973.

32. Isabel McIsaac, "Proceedings of the Fifteenth Annual Convention of the ANA," 973.

33. A Member, "Proceedings of the Fifteenth Annual Convention of the ANA," 973.

34. Mary Gladwin, "Proceedings of the Fifteenth Annual Convention of the ANA," 973–4.

35. Minnie Ahrens, "Proceedings of the Fifteenth Annual Convention of the ANA," 974.

36. Editorial Comment, "The Chicago Conventions," *AJN,* 12 no. 10 (July 1912): 769.

37. Ibid., 772.

38. Lavinia L. Dock, "Editorial Comment: The Cologne Congress," *AJN,* 12 no. 12 (September 1912): 988.

39. "Nursing News and Announcements International: Resolutions Adopted at Cologne," *AJN,* 12 no. 12 (September 1912): 1036.

40. Lavinia L. Dock, "Foreign Department: White Slavery and Legislation," *AJN,* 13 no. 3 (1912): 200.

41. Lavinia L. Dock, "Foreign Department: The Progress of Nursing in Germany," *AJN,* 13 no. 4 (January 1913): 287.

42. "Editorial Comment: Recognition of the Nursing Profession," *AJN,* 13 no. 6 (March 1913): 414.

43. "Editorial Comment: Nurses in Suffrage Parade," *AJN,* 13 no. 7 (April 1913): 489.

44. Ibid., 490.

45. Ibid.

46. Ibid., 491.

47. "Nursing News and Announcements: District of Columbia, Washington," *AJN,* 13 no. 7 (April 1913): 551.

48. "Nursing News and Announcements: Connecticut, The Hartford Hospital Training School Alumnae Association," *AJN,* 13 no. 7 (April 1913): 546. The suffrage talk was given by M. Toscan Bennett.

49. Adelaide Nutting, *Proceedings of the Nineteenth Annual Convention of the NLNE,* (Baltimore: Williams & Wilkins, 1913), 47–50; and Adelaide Nutting, "Report of the International Council of Nurses (Condensed) at the Sixteenth Annual Convention of the ANA," *AJN,* 13 no. 12 (September 1913): 940–943.

50. Mayor Riddle, Opening address presented at the sixteenth annual convention of the ANA held June 25–27, 1913, Unpublished proceedings, MML, NA, N 87, Convention Proceedings, Box 12, (no folder, in separate book), pp. 25–26.

51. Lavinia L. Dock, "Status of the Nurse in the Working World," *AJN,* 13 no. 12 (September 1913): 974.

52. Ibid.

53. George Dock, "Essentials of Professional Education," *Proceedings of the Twentieth Annual Convention of the National League of Nursing Education* (Baltimore: Williams & Wilkins Co., 1914), 76.

54. Adda Eldridge, "The Progress of the Past Year in Nursing Legislation and Some Lines of Future Effort, *Proceedings of the Twentieth Annual Convention of the National League of Nursing Education* (Baltimore: Williams & Wilkins, 1914), 93.

55. Ibid., 102.

56. Ibid.

57. Ibid., 103.

58. Ibid., 104.

59. Ibid., 105.

60. Lila Pickhardt, Recent Legislation Governing Hours of Duty of Pupil Nurses in Hospitals, *Proceedings of the Twentieth Annual Convention of the*

National League of Nursing Education (Baltimore: Williams & Wilkins, 1914), 109. Hospitals did not want a reduction of work hours for economic reasons, and some nursing leaders did not want the nursing profession to be associated with labor.

61. Seventh Annual Convention of the NACGN, August 18, 1914. Unpublished proceedings, NACGNR, Schomburg, Box 1, Volume 1, p. 68; report by a delegate Sharp of the International Congress in San Francisco at the eighth annual convention of NACGN, August 17, 1915, Unpublished proceedings, NACGNR, Schomburg, Box 1, Volume 1, p. 73.

62. Clara Noyes, *Proceedings of the Twenty-first Annual Convention of the National League of Nursing Education* (Baltimore: Williams & Wilkins, 1915), 19.

63. Ibid., 20; Clara Noyes, address by president of the National League of Nursing Education, eighteenth annual convention of the American Nurses' Association, Unpublished proceedings, MML-NA, Box 34, Folder 8, p. 38.

64. In 1915 the NLNE held its twenty-first annual convention and the ANA held its eighteenth annual convention.

65. Sara Parsons, "Report of the Publicity Committee." *Proceedings of the Twenty-first Annual Convention of the NLNE,* 75.

66. Parsons, Discussion of "Report of the Publicity Committee," *Proceedings of the Twenty-first Annual Convention of the NLNE,* 77.

67. "Miss Whitney," *Proceedings of the Twenty-first Annual Convention of the NLNE,* (Baltimore: Williams & Wilkins Co., 1915), 176–177. The proceedings do not include a full name for Miss Whitney, but she may have been suffragist speaker Anita Whitney, mentioned in Harper, *History of Woman Suffrage,* 546. Flexner, *Century of Struggle,* 274; Stevens, *Jailed for Freedom,* provides a background of the militant suffragist activities of Alice Paul; Zophy and Kavenik, *Handbook of American Women's History,* 416–418, for description of the National Woman's Party. The Congressional Union was formed in April 1913 by more militant suffragists, Alice Paul and Lucy Burns, and became the National Woman's Party.

68. "Miss Whitney," 176–177.

69. Ibid., 177.

70. Ibid., 178.

71. Kent, "Friday Morning, June 25, General Session," *AJN,* 15 no. 11 (August 1915): 1060.

72. Goodrich, "Friday Morning, June 25, General Session," 1061.

73. Taylor, "Friday Morning, June 25, General Session," 1062.

74. Effie J. Taylor, "Proceedings of the Eighteenth Annual Convention of the ANA," 1062; Effie J. Taylor, introducing the Susan B. Anthony amendment during the eighteenth annual convention of the ANA [June 1915], p. 219, Unpublished proceedings, MML-NA, N 87, Box 34, Folder 11.

75. Anna Jammé, speaking on Lavinia Dock's behalf at the eighteenth annual convention of the ANA [June 1915], p. 221. Unpublished proceedings, MML-NA, N 87, Box 34, Folder 11; and Anna Jammé, "Proceedings of the Eighteenth Annual Convention of the ANA," *AJN,* 15 no. 11, (August 1915): 1062.

76. Annie Goodrich, in a report from the president of the ICN at the eighteenth annual convention of the ANA, [1915], p. 4. Unpublished proceedings, MML-NA, N 87, Box 34, Folder 8.

77. D. Elva Stanley, "Nursing and Citizenship," *AJN,* 16 no. 1 (October 1915): 16.

78. Jeanette Waits, "The Early Years: The History of MNA 1900–1920." In *Mississippi Nurses Association Passing on the Flame: The History of the Mississippi Nurses' Association, 1911–1986* (Jackson, MS: MNA, 1986), 8–9. For a history of the woman suffrage campaign waged in Mississippi, see Harper, *The History of Woman Suffrage, 326–341.*

79. Clara Noyes, "Address," In *Proceedings of the Twenty-Second Annual Convention of the NLNE* (Baltimore: Williams & Wilkins, 1916), 21. The NLNE membership was up to 500 active members, which Noyes considered to be small in comparison with the 1,000 schools of nursing in the United States.

80. Miss Foy, "Report of the Michigan State League," *Twenty-Second Annual Convention of the NLNE,* 63–64; Alice Tarbell Crathern, *In Detroit . . . Courage Was the Fashion: The Contributions of Women to the Development of Detroit from 1701 to 1951* (Detroit: Wayne University Press, 1953), 87–88; Harper, *History of Woman Suffrage,* 303–16. Michigan State Nurses' Association, considered an active group of women, had supported woman suffrage in 1907, maintained affiliations with several women's groups, and became a member of the Federation of Women's Clubs in 1908. The State Federation of Women's Clubs, with over eight thousand members, endorsed woman suffrage in October 1908.

81. Nutting, "The Relation of the War Program to Nursing in Civil Hospitals," [read before the Twenty-fourth Annual Convention of the

NLNE, in Cleveland, Ohio, May 1918], *A Sound Economic Basis For Schools of Nursing,* 239.

82. Lavinia Dock, "Outline of Educational Conditions Internationally Considered," *Proceedings of the Twenty-third Annual Convention of the NLNE* (Baltimore: Williams & Wilkins, 1917), 120; Harper, *History of Woman Suffrage,* 756.

83. Marie Lockwood, "The Relation of the Private Duty Nurse as a Social Worker," *Proceedings of the Twenty-third Annual Convention of NLNE,* (Baltimore: Williams & Wilkins, 1917), 266.

84. Harper, *History of Woman Suffrage,* 465–8, for discussion of the victorious suffrage campaign in New York State.

85. Editorial Comment, "Miss Anthony's Vision Realized," *AJN,* 18 no. 3 (December 1917): 179–80.

86. Flexner, *Century of Struggle,* 293; Stevens, *Jailed for Freedom,* 81–90, 358. Some of the other nurses in addition to Lavinia Dock who participated in the activities of the Congressional Union and the Woman's Party and mentioned in Steven's book include Sarah Tarleton Colvin, a graduate nurse from Johns Hopkins Training School in Baltimore and a Red Cross nurse; Hattie Kruger, a trained nurse from Buffalo who worked in the Lighthouse Settlement in Philadelphia and who ran for Congress on the Socialist ticket in 1918; Mary Brown, a field nurse during the Civil War; and Mary Bartlett Dixon, a graduate of the Johns Hopkins Training School in Baltimore.

87. National League of Nursing Education Executive Board meeting minutes, May 11, 1918. [Resolutions], National League for Nursing Education Board of Directors Minutes, May 1916–June 1922 [Machine-readable date file], Unpublished minutes, NLM, HMD, NLN, MS.C. 274, Box 4, Reel 2, Bethesda.

88. Annie Goodrich (1919). "Address of Welcome," *Twenty-Fourth Annual Report of NLNE* (held in 1918), (Baltimore: Williams & Wilkins, 1919), 84–89.

89. S. Lillian Clayton, "Address of Welcome," *Proceedings of the Twenty-Fourth Annual Convention of the NLNE,* 79.

90. Helen Hoy Greeley, "Rank For Nurses," *Proceedings of the Twenty-Fourth Annual Convention of the NLNE,* 300; Lenah Sutcliff Higbee, "Nursing As It Relates to the War, *Twenty-Fourth Annual Convention of the NLNE,* 229–234; Jane A. Delano, "Nursing As It Relates To The War, *Twenty-Fourth Annual Convention of the NLNE,* 234–245; M. Adelaide Nutting, "Nursing As It Relates To The War, *Twenty-Fourth*

Annual Convention of the NLNE, 246–249; Dora Thompson, "Nursing As It Relates to the War," *Twenty-Fourth Annual Convention of the NLNE,* 226–229.

91. Helen McMillan, "Twenty-first Annual Convention of the ANA Report of the Committee on Resolutions, *AJN,* 18 no. 11 (August, 1918): 1097. Two different spellings for M. Helena McMillan, chairman of the Committee on Resolutions appear in the twenty-first annual convention proceedings in 1918: MacMillan on p. 1097 and M. Helena McMillan on p. 1098.

92. Lavinia Dock, "Foreign Department: A Woman's Peace Party," *AJN,* 16 no. 2 (1915): 665.

93. Dock, "A Woman's Peace Party," 665; C. Van Blarcom, A., Daspet, and M. Patterson, *Proceedings of the Twenty-Third Annual Convention of the NLNE,* 298–299. In 1917 the American Nurses' Association, the National League of Nursing Education, and the National Organization for Public Health Nursing sent a joint resolution supporting war prohibition in a telegram to President Woodrow Wilson.

94. McMillan, *Twenty-first Annual Convention of the American Nurses' Association,* 1097.

95. Laura Logan, Report of the Ohio State League of Nursing Education, *Twenty-Fourth Annual Report of the NLNE,* 63.

96. [First name unknown to author] McKenna, [Report of South Carolina's State League of Nursing Education], *Twenty-Fourth Annual Report of NLNE,* 66–67. The report does not clearly indicate whether the six women appointed to serve on the board were nurses.

97. Ibid., 66–67; Katherine DeWitt, Proceedings of the Twenty-first Annual Convention of the American Nurses' Association: Secretary's Report, *AJN,* 18 no. 11 (August 1918): 943–945.

98. Ira Couch Wood, "Address of Welcome," *Proceedings of the Twenty-Fifth Annual Convention of the National League of Nursing Education,* (Baltimore: Williams & Wilkins, 1919), 16; for description of state ratification of the federal suffrage amendment on June 4, 1919, in Illinois, see Harper, *History of Woman Suffrage,* 164.

99. Wood, ibid., 19; Kalisch and Kalisch, *The Advance of American Nursing,* 360–1, for a discussion of the devastating flu epidemic which lasted from September 1918 until August 1919 and had a death rate of some 548,452, five times higher than were killed in World War I; Dora E. Thompson, "How the Army Nursing Service Met the Demands of the War"; Lenah Sutcliff Higbee, "Work of the Navy Nurse Corps"; Clara

D. Noyes, "The Red Cross Nursing Service Here and Abroad"; Annie W. Goodrich, "Distribution of the Army School of Nursing," *Proceedings of the Twenty-Fifth Annual Convention NLNE*, (Baltimore: Williams & Wilkins, 1919), 117–26, 126–35, 135–46, 146–155, for discussion of the different military nurse corps.

100. Laura R. Logan, Report of the Secretary, *Proceedings of the Twenty-Fifth Annual Convention of the NLNE*, 27–32.

101. Helen Hoy Greeley, Anna Maxwell, and Clara Noyes, [Discussion of war and post-war activities relating to nursing] *Proceedings of the Twenty-Fifth Annual Convention of the National League of Nursing Education*, (Baltimore: Williams & Wilkins, 1919), 190–96.

102. Report of Adah Thoms Opening Address, Twelfth Annual Convention of the National Association of Colored Graduate Nurses, August 19, 1919, Unpublished proceedings of the NACGN, Schomburg, Box 1, Volume 2, pp. 64–65.

103. Laura Rebekah Logan [Discussion on membership], *Proceedings of the Twenty-Sixth Annual Convention of the National League of Nursing Education* (held in 1920) (Baltimore: Williams & Wilkins, 1921), 198.

104. Anna Jammé [Discussion on membership], *Proceedings of the Twenty-Sixth Annual Convention of the NLNE*, 189–203.

105. W. P. Morril, "School of Nurses with University Affiliation," *Proceedings of the Twenty-Sixth Annual Convention of the NLNE*, 303.

106. For Nutting's views on woman suffrage, see Marshall, *Mary Adelaide Nutting: Pioneer of Modern Nursing* (Baltimore: Johns Hopkins Press, 1972); Adelaide Nutting, *The Outlook in Nursing, Proceedings of the Twenty-Sixth Annual Convention of the National League of Nursing Education* (held in 1920), (Baltimore: Williams & Wilkins, 1921), 309–10.

107. Flexner, *Century of Struggle*, 336–37, for discussion of the final victory for the federal suffrage amendment; Burgess, *Nurses, Patients, and Pocketbooks*, 61. There were an estimated 150,000 practicing nurses in 1920.

5

Taking Charge

We have been, until very recently, lifting our voices to the deaf ears of ignorance and prejudice concerning the most fundamental principles of sense and justice as related to the education and practice of nurses.

Sara Parsons, 1920[1]

WINNING THE VOTE in 1920 meant that women could exercise political control in their personal and professional lives. The franchise signified the woman movement's success in propelling women from the narrowly defined prescribed roles in the home into the more autonomous self-determined roles outside. By the second decade of the twentieth century, the woman's sphere had extended into the world of education, work, and suffrage. No longer was there just one role for women, and although custom and paternalistic bias in society still restrained them, the law sanctioned women equal by virtue of the Nineteenth Amendment. After 1920, women could partake in all elections; ergo, they could politically represent their own interests in their own voice.

While the woman movement challenged women's roles, the modern nursing movement, beginning in 1873, transformed the "natural" woman's role of nursing into a professional role: one that demanded education, knowledge, and self-determination. Late nineteenth-century women seminaries and colleges educated women to assume their rightful roles of wife, mother, and teacher and promised the nation better prepared moral guardians of family life. However, the new schools did not prepare them to take on an even greater role specifically assigned to women: the role of nurse. Consequently, following Florence Nightingale's successful use of educated nurses, women's education in America included the education of nurses.

Nursing education provided women an opportunity to be self-supporting as well as the opportunity to move out of a sphere of domesticity and into a sphere of "action."[2] Nursing schools emancipated women and gave them "a chance to grow."[3] Nursing, specifically as intended by the early nursing pioneers such as Nightingale, challenged the limited boundaries of women's work and may have equally questioned the domestic feminists ideas of the moral superiority of women's work. Nightingale specified that gender should not determine the worth of a job when she explained that "it does not make a thing good, that it is remarkable that a woman should have been able to do it. Neither does it make a thing bad, which would have been good had a man done it, that it has been done by a woman."[4]

The domestic feminism of the nineteenth century gave way to the social feminists in the late nineteenth and early twentieth century, and educated women supported various social reform movements of the Progressive Era. The settlement house movement, the public health movement, and the modern nursing movement found women activists ready to improve the health and well-being of society. Women formed organizations to do some of the social housekeeping activities required of them to improve society. The nineteenth- and early twentieth-century women's organizations that formed provided women a means to release their political energies and their intellectual drive.

The modern nursing movement, however, uniquely provided not only opportunities to improve society, but availed women an education and paid employment for work that had social significance. The nursing organizations which formed during the late nineteenth and early twentieth century differed from other newly formed organized women's groups because for the first time women organized for professional growth and control. Nurses applied social feminist activism to their own professional needs to ensure the health of society. In their clinical practice, nurses poignantly saw firsthand the political connection between improved health and their own political involvement. Consequently, nurses moved from the parochial concern of establishing a neophyte profession to embrace a global interest in the world around them.

As the woman movement sought political equality for women, nursing leaders argued for professional equality for nursing. The modern nursing movement cultivated women's intellectual drive and ability to financially support themselves and to participate in social reform activities. Through the establishment of nurse training schools and organized nursing associations, nurses could articulate professional goals and politically aspire to achieve these goals within their organizations.

The right of "voting in political matters, or the exercise of that right; especially in a representative form of government" defined suffrage; the vote gave women personal suffrage, or the right to exercise the vote in political matters that pertained to personal freedom.[5] Nurses too enjoyed the personal freedom that suffrage would bring. Yet prior to the 1920s' federal suffrage victory, nurses exercised a form of professional suffrage within their nursing organizations. Whether in local nurse training school alumnae associations, state associations, or national associations, nurses voted within these organizations on matters concerning their education, practice, and livelihood. However, in spite of their professional suffrage, personal suffrage would not fully emerge until women obtained the vote in 1920; only then were nurses finally able to vote for legislation that would enhance their profession.

The woman suffrage issue emerged as both a professional and a pragmatic concern for American nurses. Nursing had exercised a practical feminism, or nurses' rights feminism, for years; thus, support of the woman suffrage movement was a logical conclusion. If feminism is, as defined by turn of the century writer Alice Duer Miller's (1874–1942) poetry: "A Feminist, my daughter, is any woman now who cares to think about her own affairs as men don't think she ougher," then the practical feminism in nursing directed nursing's feminist activities toward taking charge of its own affairs as many in the paternalistic health care system did not think it ougher. The nursing organizations in America declared their interest in the study of woman suffrage in 1908 and officially sanctioned their support in 1912. The woman's vote was viewed as imperative for nurses to access political control of the profession's development in the world outside of the profession.[6] As one English nurse in 1915 noted at a nursing convention in San Francisco, American nurses had achieved professional enfranchisement far ahead of their English colleagues.[7]

With the founding of the International Council of Nurses (ICN) in 1899, nurses throughout the world united their efforts to establish a recognized "system of nursing education" and to gain "control over the nursing profession." Only through unified action could nurses hope to be of utmost usefulness in their work with the sick, argued the originator of the ICN, Ethel Gordon Fenwick, in 1901. Fenwick explained that the first aim of the ICN was to organize nurses into professional organizations where they could develop "corporate responsibility" for the profession. Fenwick continued, "thus, in the formation of national councils of federations of nurses *graduate suffrage* must ultimately be adopted as a fundamental principle." Through the graduate nurses' vote, professional control over the standards for nursing education and the setting of qualifications for trained nurses could be accomplished. Decisions about education and qualifications had to be established among the graduate trained nurses before nursing could "demand legal status." Fenwick described a "Nursing Tree" where delegates from the ICN would encourage the formation of alumnae associations, national associations, and national councils which relied on the graduate nurses' vote in order to unify nursing's activity and secure state registration.[8]

To this end, woman suffrage emerged as pivotal to advancing nurses' professional goals, nationally and internationally. Evidence of American nursing's interest in suffrage can be seen in the seven times that organizations voted on whether to support woman suffrage, as well as the more than 200 times that woman suffrage appeared in its papers, speeches, published articles, and letters to the editor. Hence, every nurse who was a member of one of the professional nursing organizations, or who read one of the nursing journals, participated in the suffrage debate.

From the founding of the Superintendents' Society in 1893 until the founding of the National Organization for Public Health Nursing (NOPHN) in 1912, nursing had steadily moved from tending to the details of establishing a new profession to expanding its professional horizons to include the global issues confronting nurses and all women in society. Like other woman suffragists, many nurses wanted to control their own destiny through exercising their right to vote.

Many of the nursing leaders of the Superintendents' Society, the Associated Alumnae, and the NOPHN shared a pro-suffrage sentiment and believed that the only way to convince other nurses of the importance of the vote was through intensive education. Thus, the frequency of suffrage references resulted from the active educative roles played by the organizations to enlighten their memberships on woman's rights. Topics that provided nurses with the intellectual link between nursing and suffrage varied. Nurse registration in each state provided nurses with a strong rationale to support woman suffrage; the daily health care problems faced by public health nurses in urban and rural settings supplied additional arguments to support suffrage, and nursing's constant struggle to control educational standards, working hours of student nurses, central nursing directories, military rank for nurses, and social reforms further influenced nursing's opinion on suffrage legislation. Thus, the striking issues confronting the profession and society convinced nurses of the efficacy of the franchise. Consequently, nursing's campaign to educate nurses to this vital issue linked the vote to the health of society and the future advancement of the nursing profession. For nurses, the ability to vote was directly related to the idea of professional suffrage.

In the quest to control nursing through woman suffrage, nursing organizations sought the shared experiences of other women's groups. Nursing's early affiliation with the National Council of Women (NCW), the International Council of Women (ICW), and the International Council of Nurses (ICN) recognized the mutual concerns nurses and other women faced in a worldwide struggle for political freedom. Women's organizations and professional nursing organizations advocated women's rights and in most instances strongly supported woman suffrage. The Superintendents' Society, Associated Alumnae, NACGN, and NOPHN affiliations with other women's associations illustrated nursing's collaboration with others interested in obtaining women's rights. Nursing's compelling need to command and guard its own profession defined the extent of American nursing's participation in the suffrage campaign.

The modern nursing movement paralleled other exciting world movements during the Progressive Era: suffrage, prohibition, moral prophylaxis, and peace movements flourished in the hands of woman reformers. Adelaide Nutting told American Federation of Nurses' delegates in 1909 how reform movements had influenced nursing's development and needed nursing's support. Nutting considered woman suffrage as one of the greatest movements of the day and one which nurses should promote. Nurses could no longer remain ignorant of the suffrage issue and no matter what one's personal views were regarding this subject, nurses professionally had to become more knowledgeable.[9]

In 1909, Linna Richardson spoke of the interrelationship between nursing and society, which required political savvy to maintain. While nursing advanced its own professional cause to improve humanity, humanity, would in turn assist the nursing profession to advance. Richardson predicted that the profession's interest in state nurse registration and central nursing registries would find friends among the other reform movements which nursing supported. She envisioned that the successful nurse of the future would be sufficiently wise and broad-minded to realize the significance of collaborative efforts with other reform groups for the professional maturation of nursing.[10]

As the woman suffrage movement intensified its campaign in 1912, nurses in the ANA voted to support an organizational woman suffrage resolution. Once agreed on, the ANA sent four delegates to the ICN Congress in Germany that year who were prepared to support an international woman suffrage resolution. This action historically cemented the relationship between the modern nursing movement and the woman suffrage movement. Yet, in spite of professional nursing organizations' interest in and support of woman's rights documented by records of the organizations, the numerous discussions and articles published by articulate nursing suffragist Lavinia Dock and others, until recently, all have been forgotten. The 1908 defeat of nursing's support of woman suffrage at the Associated Alumnae Convention in San Francisco often epitomized nursing's relationship with the woman's movement. Nursing has been labeled as historically conservative and the events of the 1908 suffrage vote seen as indicative of nursing's rejection of the woman's movement. Nurse historian Jo Ann Ashley explained, "to the detriment of their own growth as professional persons, nurses were among the most conservative of conservatives."[11]

However, such descriptions of nursing's role within the late nineteenth and early twentieth century reflect a limited interpretation of nursing's activities. Rather than unsupportive, the vote in 1908 reflected an increasing interest among nurses in the suffrage question; defeat of organizational support illustrated the demand for broadening nurses' understanding of suffrage, and the ensuing educational campaign following the defeat suggested nurses' strong interest in issues outside of their professional practice. The successful passage of organizational support of suffrage by 1912 and the additional resolutions that followed sealed nursing's relationship with the woman suffrage movement.

The efforts following the 1908 vote by women who linked nurses' professional role and social responsibility to the woman's movement at large must be acknowledged. In their efforts for professional self-determination in education and practice, nurses faced paternalistic impediments along the way. To oppose such restraints on professional freedom, nurses supported political freedom and played an important role within the woman movement.

Nursism

In spite of nursing's role in the woman suffrage movement, the gnawing presence of the devalued role of the nursing profession persists into the late twentieth century. The nursing profession has fallen prey to the insidious ideology of nursism: a form of sexism that specifically maligns the caring role in society. Sexism refers to the subordinate social position in which women have been placed. Although the term "sexism" has been used frequently in the latter half of the twentieth century by the women's movement, sexism had existed long before. Keeping women as unenfranchised citizens historically demonstrates one of the more blatant forms of sexism that women had to endure and overcome. However, other more insidious forms of sexism exist that control and belittle the role of women in society. For example, language that reflects sexist values, as seen in the frequently used term "man" as generic for people, tends to erode women's worth in society.[12] Assigning monetary value to work based on roles specifically designated to gender illustrates another devastating form of sexism. The pervasive spread of sexism that artificially divides activities into women's work or men's work can be better described using the term "nursism," explaining the societal value placed on the caring role of the nurse.[13]

Since the late nineteenth and early twentieth century, the nursing profession has been labeled a predominantly female profession. Not only were women considered naturally suited to nursing, but the caring role itself "naturally" belonged within the women's sphere. Throughout the modern nursing movement, the caring role, practiced by nursing, has been subordinate to the curing role, practiced by physicians.[14]

Thus, nursism negatively influenced the development of the nursing profession and possibly was what impelled Superintendents' Society President Mary Riddle in 1911 to question how educated women would be attracted to nursing, a profession which was so often forgotten, or remembered with dread. Riddle poignantly asked:

> *how the educated young woman may be interested in this work of ours which is paradoxical in offering so much and so little—so much of opportunity for usefulness, and so little in worldly advancement.*[15]

Although the nursing profession offered women work in what was perceived as a woman's occupation and thus considered less threatening to men, nursing nevertheless faced paternalistic control. For the most part, men feared financial, emotional, and social loss of power from women who marched for woman rights or worked in typically male-defined occupations. Early twentieth-century writer Alice Duer Miller satirically illustrated the feelings expressed by men who feared loss of jobs and subsequently passed laws prohibiting women from working in them. In her poem, "The Gallant Sex," Miller referred to the case of a woman engineer who lost her job because the board of education passed a rule that women should not work with high pressure boilers:

> Lady, dangers lurk in boilers,
>   risks I could not let you face.
> Men were meant to be the toilers,
>   Home, you know is woman's place.
> Have no home? Well, is that so?
>   Still, it's not my fault, you know.
> Charming lady, work no more;
>   Fair you are and sweet as honey;
> Work might make your fingers sore,
>   And, besides, I need the money.
> Prithee rest,—or starve or rob—
> Only let me have your job![16]

While few men entered nursing, the closing line for a similar poem for nurses might have been written instead as, ". . . only let me tell you how to do your job." Discrimination rested not in women encroaching on men's private sphere of influence, but rather in a paternalistic society wanting to control all spheres, especially women's work. While women were discriminated against by virtue of their gender, nurses were discriminated against by virtue of the role that they undertook, regardless of their gender. As a result, nurses had to spend tremendous energy overcoming this form of prejudice: to convince educated women to enter the profession, to convince those coming into the profession to be educated, and to convince society of the need to educate nurses.[17]

At the outset of the modern nursing movement, Florence Nightingale attempted to elevate the public's perception of nursing from the Sairey Gamp image toward the idea "that nursing was an art, and must be raised to the status of a trained profession."[18] Nurse training schools that began in 1873 with the ideals imparted by Nightingale aspired to self-determination. Twenty years later, nursing organizations formed to improve existing schools and assert a controlling interest in nursing.

All of the nursing organizations that formed between 1893 and 1920 concerned themselves with perpetuation of the profession through fresh new recruits in nurse training schools. In 1915, the NLNE spoke of its efforts to recruit nursing students, and through its vocational guidance committee studied the reasons why some women did not select nursing as a career. The committee learned that women did not enter the profession because of "the nature of many of the prejudices against nursing which many people tell us are pretty firmly fixed in the popular mind."[19]

According to the vocational guidance committee's findings, the average high school girl had ". . . a very lively sense of the horrors and tragedies which the public generally associates with nursing work." Some additional reasons for not selecting nursing were: nurses would not meet the right kind of people, nurses were not respected, candidates were unsure if they had the physical strength required of the job, and parental disapproval of nursing. The results of the study also suggested that the underlying misconceptions of and prejudices against nursing had to be addressed before young women would be attracted into nursing. Nursing educator Isabel Stewart pointedly explained that until nursing was better understood, there would be little appreciation of nursing's work and it would be difficult to recruit a sufficient number of high school girls to the profession.

Stewart, who presented the vocational guidance committee report, identified the advantages to nursing that respondents had listed. The positive reasons women entered the nursing profession included: educational advantages, development of one's own powers, opportunities for personal and community service, special interests and satisfactions, economic advantages leading to financial independence, and positive effect on home and family. However, almost twenty years after the founding of the organizations and five years after Stewart's vocational guidance committee report, former NLNE president Sara Parsons (1917–1918) looked back at nursing traditions of obedience and devotion and reflected how they had created "a very real handicap." Paraphrasing Nightingale, who said that no man or physician ever gave a definition for nurses other than "devoted and obedient," Parsons felt this paternalistic definition might have done for a horse, but would not have done for a policeman. The traditions of devotion and obedience in nursing had taken on a "lamentable shackling effect," which she hoped to be delivered from; nursing had been " 'devoted and obedient' to the point of complete subordination to medical authority and custom." Nurses who tried to explain to the public what was needed in nursing education found their explanations had fallen on "the deaf ears of ignorance and prejudice concerning the fundamental principles of sense and justice as related to the education and practice of nurses."[20] In a speech Parsons delivered at the twenty-third annual convention of the NLNE held in Philadelphia in April 1917, she exclaimed that "if ever a profession had to contend with misunderstanding, misrepresentation, antagonism, and exploitation, it's nursing."[21]

The image of nursing hinged a great deal on society's preconceived notions of women's work and the value society placed on that work. Nursing education, the key to the advancement of the profession, received limited public support as nursing educators tried to move nurse training from the outdated hospital apprenticeship mode of education into colleges and universities. The first college to prepare trained nurses opened in 1911 at the University of Minnesota. However, the collegiate movement in nursing began with little financial support and much opposition to the "overeducated" nurse. Therefore, due to the persistent stereotypical ideal of the "born nurse" and misconceptions of the knowledge base in art and science required in nursing practice, the collegiate movement was slow to develop or significantly advance nursing education at the baccalaureate level.[22]

Nursing organizations worked diligently to overcome the nursisms that hindered the advancement of nursing education and limited the control of nursing practice. Political enfranchisement was seen as the means to empower nurses to accomplish their professional and personal goals. However, even after the profession supported woman suffrage, and even after woman suffrage was granted, the myths and misconceptions promoting sexism and nursism did not disappear from American life. It remained a backdrop throughout the twentieth century and has continued through the 1990s to restrain women and the profession of nursing from taking on a more equal role in society.

The resurgence of the women's movement in the late 1960s, while promoting the advancement of women in male defined professions, ignored the political, professional, and personal possibilities women created in the profession of nursing.[23] The women's movement did not know of or recognize nursing's historical ties with the woman movement at the beginning of the twentieth century. It could only see the glaring inequity in rank, social status, and economic reward between practitioners in medicine and in nursing. Even the theoretical underpinning of nursing science necessary for an emerging profession had been undervalued, "unacknowledged, trivialized when compared to medicine as the more mature science." Nursing has been "considered as incidental, therefore less valuable to successful treatment when compared to more dramatic medical intervention."[24] The result encouraged few women and even fewer men to enter the profession of nursing.

The feminine role associated with nursing has been placed in a subordinate position and has been omitted as a valued role in society. Both the activities associated with nurses' work and the political control by physicians and hospital administrators over nursing activities have contributed to nursing's perceived powerlessness in society. Nursing and nurses, using little of their power generated within the historical context, seem to embody the very characteristics and problems that many contemporary feminists have challenged. Consequently, some nursing leaders speculate that feminists have "failed to look beyond the inaccurate, sexist stereotypes of nurses to even acknowledge the multiple dimensions of professional nursing."[25] Yet, paradoxically, nursing has been described by others as a metaphor for the ". . . struggle of women for equality."[26]

Since the 1970s, nursing literature has begun to reflect nursing's renewed identification with women's issues, specifically those issues exemplified by the women's movement and feminism.[27] Women's historian Susan Reverby argued that contemporary feminism served to give ". . . nursing a political language that stresses equality and rights within the given order of things."[28] Nurses today have begun to recognize and challenge the devastating political, social, and economic effects sexism has had on nurses and on women health care consumers. As a result, nursing and nursing knowledge have begun to be studied, taught, and practiced using a feminist framework. Furthermore, there has been a growing recognition of the similarity between women's history and nursing's history. That similarity has prompted investigations into the relationship between them.[29]

Newer paradigms for nursing education, practice, and research reflect a feminist framework that is rooted in the history of the profession. The early woman movement found support, "solidarity . . . and great loyalty," from the nursing profession.[30] The prejudice accepted by society and displayed toward the caring role of the nurse has been regarded as customary for too long and is still not sufficiently challenged. However, an exploration of nursism uncovers nursing's rich history and challenges nursing's invisible and stereotypical image. Nursing must recover its social history, turn to its pioneering leaders as mentors, use the hard won vote in the political arena, and challenge the nursism that surrounds the profession of nursing. Only in this way will nursing be able to attract women and men into the field and provide the humanistic health care society will require in the next century.[31]

NOTES

1. Sara E. Parsons, "What Teachers College Means to an Old Alumna," "Twenty-Five Years of Nursing Education in Teachers College 1899–1925," *Teachers College Bulletin,* 17th series no. 3 (February 1926): 45. Parsons was an alumna of Teachers College from the class of 1904–5 and first read her paper at the twentieth anniversary of the department of nursing in 1920.

2. Stewart, *The Education of Nurses,* 47.

3. Ibid., 78.

4. Nightingale, *Notes on Nursing,* 135–6.

5. William Allan Neilson, Thomas Knott, and Paul Carhart, eds., *Webster's New International Dictionary of the English Language,* 2nd ed., unabridged

(Springfield, MA: G. and C. Merriam Company, 1939), 2520, provides a definition of suffrage.

6. Wald, "The Nurses' Settlement," *Sixth Annual Convention of the ASSTSN,* 55–57.

7. Kent, "Friday Morning, June 25, General Session," *AJN,* 15 no. 11 (August 1915): 1060.

8. Ethel Gordon Fenwick, "The International Council of Nurses, A Message from the President," *AJN,* 1 no. 11 (August 1901): 787–9.

9. Nutting, President's Opening Remarks at the Second Meeting of the AFN, *Fifteenth Annual Report of ASSTN including Report of the Second Meeting of the AFN, 1909,* 106.

10. Richardson, "Reasons for Central Registries and Club Houses, *Proceedings of the Twelfth Annual Convention of the ANA,* 984.

11. Ashley, "Nurses in American History Nursing and Early Feminism," 1465; Peggy Chinn, "Historical Roots: Female Nurses and Political Action," *The Journal of the New York Nurses Association,* 16 no. 2 (June 1985): 29–37; Teresa Christy, "Equal Rights for Women: Voice from the Past," *Pages From Nursing History: A Collection of Original Articles from the Pages of Nursing Outlook, The American Journal of Nursing and Nursing Research* (New York: American Journal of Nursing, 1984), 64; Mary Ellen Doona, "Nursing Revisited: Memories—Armistice and Suffrage," *The Massachusetts Nurse,* 52 no. 11 (November 1983): 15, for discussion of the 1908 anti-suffrage vote; Charlene Eldridge Wheeler, "The American Journal of Nursing and the Socialization of a Profession," *Advance in Nursing Science,* 7 no. 2 (January 1985): 20–34, presents nursing's "solidarity with and great loyalty to the cause of women's progress," between 1900 and 1920 and discusses the nursing organizations' change in neutral policy toward support of suffrage by 1913.

12. Peggy Chinn, "Historical Roots: Female Nurses and Political Action," 29–37, for a discussion of the effect of sexism in nursing; Bonnie G. Smith, "Sexism," Zophy and Kavenik, *Handbook of American Women's History,* 543, for a definition of sexism.

13. Lewenson, *The Relationship Among the Four Professional Nursing Organizations and Woman Suffrage: 1893–1920,* 179–181; Lewenson, "The Woman's Nursing and Suffrage Movement, 1893–1920," 131–132.

14. Choon and Skevington, "How Do Women and Men in Nursing Perceive Each Other?" 101–111; Heide, "Nursing and Women's Liberation: A Parallel," 824–827, Janet Muff, ed. (1982). *Socialization, Sexism, and Stereotyping,* presents numerous papers on the influence of sexism on the

nursing profession; Patricia Moccia, "Response to Women's Talk and Nurse-Client Encounters: Developing Criteria for Assessing Interpersonal Skill," *Scholarly Inquiry for Nursing Practice: An International Journal,* 1 no. 3 (1987): 257–261.

15. Mary Riddle, "President's Address," *Proceedings of the Seventeenth Annual Convention of the ASSTSN* (Baltimore: J.H. Furst Company, 1911), 22.

16. Alice Duer Miller, *Are Women People? A Book of Rhymes for Suffrage Times* (New York: George H. Doran Company, n.d.), 19.

17. Ashley, *Hospitals, Paternalism, and the Role of the Nurse,* 75–93, for discussion regarding medical opposition to advancements in nurse education.

18. Cook, *Life of Florence Nightingale,* 1:445; Bullough, Bullough, and Stanton, eds., *Florence Nightingale and Her Era: A Collection of New Scholarship,* for readings on Nightingale's influence on the modern nursing movement.

19. Isabel Stewart, "Report of the Vocational Guidance Committee," *Proceedings of the Twenty-first Annual Convention of the National League of Nursing Education,* (Baltimore: Williams & Wilkins, 1915), 47.

20. Sara Parsons, "What Teachers College Means to an Old Alumna," *Twenty-Five Years of Nursing Education 1899–1925,* 44–45.

21. Sara Parsons, "Address," *Proceedings of the Twenty-third Annual Convention of the NLNE* (Baltimore: Williams and Wilkins, 1917), 56.

22. Ashley, *Hospitals, Paternalism, and the Role of the Nurse,* 126–128, reference to the 1965 ANA's first position paper calling for the minimum education for nurses to the baccalaureate degree. Unfortunately in the 1990s, nursing has not succeeded in establishing a college degree as a basic requirement for entrance into nursing. Most nurses enter with a two-year associate degree rather than the four years required for a baccalaureate degree, and some still enter the profession with only hospital training school experience. No matter which educational route is taken into nursing, new graduates sit for the same licensing exams.

23. Mary Madeline Rogge, "Nursing and Politics: A Forgotten Legacy," *Nursing Research,* 36, no. 1 (January/February 1987): 26.

24. Moccia, "Response to 'Women's Talk' and Nurse-Client Encounters," 258.

25. L. Fitzpatrick, "Nursing," *Signs,* 2 no. 4 (1977): 818–834; Vance, Talbott, McBride, and Mason, "Coming of Age: The Women's Movement and Nursing," *Political Action Handbook for Nurses,* eds. Diana Mason and Susan W. Talbott (Menlo Park, CA: Addison Wesley, 1985), 24.

26. Donna Diers, "To Profess—To Be a Professional," 23, for nursing as a metaphor; Ruth Simmons and Jane Rosenthal, "The Women's Movement

and the Nurse Practitioner's Sense of Role," *Nursing Outlook,* 29 no. 6 (June 1981): 371–375.

27. Alice Baumgart and Rondalyn Kirkwood, "Social Reform Versus Education Reform: University Nursing Education in Canada. 1919–1960," *Journal of Advanced Nursing,* 15 (1990): 510–516; Allen, "Women, Nursing and Feminism: An Interview With Alice J. Baumgart, RN, PhD.," 20–22; Andrist, "A Feminist Framework for Graduate Education in Women's Health," 66–67; Charleston Faculty Practice Group, "Nursing Faculty Collaboration Viewed Through Feminist Process," *Advances in Nursing Science,* 8 no. 2 (January 1986): 29–38; Heide, "Nursing and Women's Liberation a Parallel," 824–827; Wilma Scott Heide, *Feminism for the Health of It,* (Buffalo, NY: Margaretdaughters, 1985); Simmons and Rosenthal, "The Women's Movement and the Nurse Practitioner's Sense of Role," 371–375; McBride, "A Married Feminist," 754–757; Starr, "Poor Baby: The Nurse and Feminism," 20–22; Talbott and Vance, "Involving Nursing in a Feminist Group—Now," 592–595.

28. Reverby, *Ordered to Care,* 207.

29. Andrist, "A Feminist Framework For Graduate Education in Women's Health," 66–70; Rosemary Amason Bowman and Rebecca Clark Culpepper, "Power: Rx for Change," *AJN* 74 no. 6 (June 1974): 1053–1056; Bonnie Bullough, "Influences on Role Expansion, *AJN,* 76 no. 9 (September 1976): 1478; Charleston Faculty Practice Group, "Nursing Faculty Collaboration Viewed Through Feminist Process," 311; Chinn and Wheeler, "Feminism and Nursing," 74–77; Virginia Cleland, "Sex Discrimination: Nursing's Most Pervasive Problem," *AJN* 71 no. 8 (August 1971): 1542–1547; Moccia, "Response to 'Women's Talk' and Nurse-Client Encounters: Developing Criteria for Assessing Interpersonal Skill," 257–261; Mary Ann Ruffing-Rahal, "Incorporating Feminism Into the Graduate Curriculum," *Nursing Education,* 31 no. 6 (June 1992): 247–252.

30. Wheeler, "The American Journal of Nursing and the Socialization of a Profession 1900–1920," 33.

31. Pamela Maraldo, "NLN's First Century," *Nursing and Health Care,* 13 no. 5 (May 1992): 227–228. Maraldo is the former chief executive officer of the National League for Nursing. Her editorial validates this author's perceptions of nursing's rich social past and its potential future contributions.

Appendix A

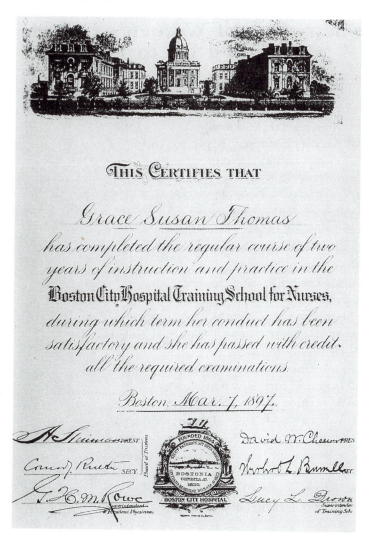

THIS CERTIFIES THAT

Grace Susan Thomas

*has completed the regular course of two
years of instruction and practice in the*
Boston City Hospital Training School for Nurses,
*during which term her conduct has been
satisfactory and she has passed with credit
all the required examinations.*

Boston, Mar. 7, 1897.

Appendix B

Sampling of Women's Groups Formed Up to 1920

National Women's Relief Society	*1842*
National Women's Christian Temperance Union	*1874*
American Association of University Women	*1882*
The Daughters of the King	*1885*
Daughters of Union Veterans of the Civil War—1861–1865	*1885*
The Needlework Guild of American	*1885*
American Physical Education Association	*1886*
Child Study Association of America	*1888*
National Council of Women	*1888*
International Council of Women	*1888*
General Federation of Women's Clubs	*1889*
Rhode Island Council of Women	*1889*
National Association of Women Painters and Sculptors	*1889*
Colonial Dames of American	*1890*
National Association of Colored Women	*1896*
National League of American Pen Women	*1897*
National Association of Women Lawyers	*1898*
National Women's Trade Union League of America	*1903*
American Home Economics Association	*1908*
Council of Women for Home Missions	*1908*
National Kindergarten Association	*1909*
National Federation of Settlements, Inc.	*1911*
Family Welfare Association of America	*1911*
Camp Fire Girls, Inc.	*1912*

Sampling of Women's Groups Formed Up to 1920

Girl Scouts, Inc.	*1912*
Federation of Women's Boards of Foreign Missions of North America	*1912*
National Women's Party	*1913*
National Motion Picture League	*1913*
National Federation of Temple Sisterhoods	*1913*
Woman's National Farm and Garden Association	*1914*
National Council of Administrative Women in Education	*1915*
National Association of Deans of Women	*1916*
National Association of Altrusa Clubs	*1917*
Big Brother and Big Sister Federation, Inc.	*1917*
Service Star Legion	*1917*
National Federation of Business and Professional Women's Clubs	*1919*
Association of Women in Public Health	*1920*
National League for Women Voters	*1920*
Osteopathic Women's National Association	*1920*

Appendix C

Nursing Organizations and Affiliations with Women's Councils

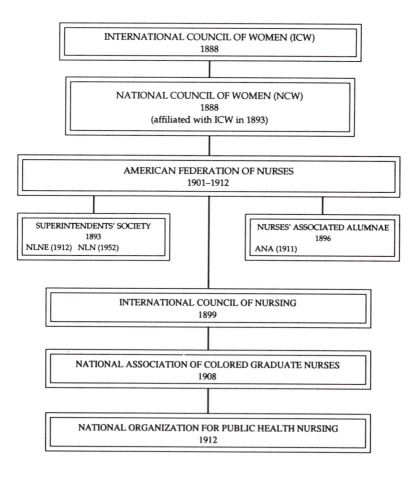

INTERNATIONAL COUNCIL OF WOMEN (ICW)
1888

NATIONAL COUNCIL OF WOMEN (NCW)
1888
(affiliated with ICW in 1893)

AMERICAN FEDERATION OF NURSES
1901–1912

SUPERINTENDENTS' SOCIETY
1893
NLNE (1912)   NLN (1952)

NURSES' ASSOCIATED ALUMNAE
1896
ANA (1911)

INTERNATIONAL COUNCIL OF NURSING
1899

NATIONAL ASSOCIATION OF COLORED GRADUATE NURSES
1908

NATIONAL ORGANIZATION FOR PUBLIC HEALTH NURSING
1912

Appendix D

of the *Johns Hopkins Hospital* *187*

Dear Miss *Hampton*

You are cordially invited to attend the first annual meeting of "The American Society of Superintendents of Training Schools for Nurses," to be held on January 10th and 11th, 1894, in this City. Three sessions will be held in Room 37, in the Academy of Medicine, No. 19 West 43d Street, at 10 A.M. and 2 P.M. on Wednesday, and at 10 A.M. on Thursday. Arrangements for board in advance may be made by writing to the Ashland House, cor. 4th Ave. and 24th Street ; or to the Margaret Louisa Home of the Y. W. C. A., 14 East 16th Street. Rates at the former place are from $2.00 to $3.00 per day ; at the latter, $1.50 per day ; rooms without board can be had, respectively, for $1.00 and 50 cts. The Grand Central Hotel, opposite the Grand Central Station, 42d Street, will accommodate guests without any preliminary arrangements at $1.00 dollar per day or upward, for rooms on the European plan.

After the necessary business of organizing has been gone through with, subjects of interest and importance to the nursing profession will be discussed in the order in which they are introduced, and it is hoped that a large and enthusiastic company will be assembled.

The Superintendents' Association, which it is hoped the approaching Convention will regularly inaugurate to meet yearly, was begun last Summer at Chicago, where, at a meeting of Superintendents, the following resolutions regarding the aim of such a society, and qualifications for membership, were drawn up, submitted and approved.

Name and Object.

(a) This Society shall be known as the American Society of Superintendents of Training Schools for Nurses.

(b) Its object shall be to promote fellowship of members ; to establish and maintain a universal standard of training ; to further the best interests of the nursing profession.

Qualifications for Membership.

(a) Members shall be graduates in good and regular standing from Training Schools connected with General Hospitals giving not less than a two years' course of instruction.

(b) Members shall be Superintendents of Training Schools, connected with recognized General Hospitals, giving not less than a two years' course of instruction.

A temporary committee, composed of Miss Alston, New York ; Miss Davis, Philadelphia ; Miss Palmer, Washington ; Miss Darche, New York ; Miss Drown, Boston ; Miss Hampton, Baltimore ; and Miss Sutliffe, New York, was selected to draft a constitution to be presented at the first meeting of the Society, January 10th, 1894.

Trusting that on this day we may have the pleasure of both seeing you and hearing you, I am,

Very truly yours,

ANNA L. ALSTON,
President pro tem.

LOUISE DARCHE,
Secretary pro tem.,
110 West 43d Street.

R.S.V.P.

Appendix E

Officers for next Annual Meeting
appointed or elected Jany 11th 1894.

President. — Miss Linda Richards, Supt. New England Hospital
Training School, Roxbury, Mass.

Vice Prest. — Miss Irene Sutliffe, Supt. Training School
New York Hospital, New York.

Secretary — Miss Mary Littlefield, Supt. Tr. School
Episcopal Hospital, Philadelphia.

Treasurer — Miss L. L. Drown, Supt. of Tr. School
Boston City Hospital, Boston

Auditors {
Miss D. C. Kimber, Ass't Supt. N. Y. City Tr.
School, Blackwell's Isld. New York.

Miss Ida Sutliffe, Supt. Long Isld. College
Hosp. Tr. Sch. Brooklyn, N. Y.
}

Councillors {
Miss I. A. Hampton, J. H. H. Baltimore, Md.
" M. I. Merritt, Bklyn Hosp. Brooklyn N. Y.
" Livingston, Montreal Gel. Hosp. Montreal, Ca.
" Maxwell, Presbyterian Hosp. New York.
Dick, 304 House St. Chicago — Ill School
Snively, Toronto Genl. Hosp. Toronto Ca
}

The 2nd. Annual Convention to be held
in Boston, 2nd. Week in February 1895.

Appendix F

Timeline: Woman Movement

1820	Florence Nightingale born May 12
1837	Mount Holyoke, first American women's college
1848	Seneca Falls Convention
1854–1856	Florence Nightingale during the Crimean War
1859	Florence Nightingale's *Notes on Nursing* published in England
1860	Nightingale School established at St. Thomas's Hospital in England
1861–1865	American Civil War
1865	Vassar College opens
1869	National Woman Suffrage Association, led by Elizabeth Cady Stanton (1815–1893) and Susan B. Anthony
	American Woman Suffrage Association, led by Henry Ward Beecher and Lucy Stone
1875	Wellesley College opens
1884	Bryn Mawr College opens
1889	Barnard College at Columbia University
1890	National American Woman Suffrage Association
1894	Radcliffe College opens at Harvard University
1914	Congressional Union for Woman Suffrage, later known as the Woman's Party

Appendix G

Timeline: Modern Nursing Movement

1879	Mary Eliza Mahoney graduated from the New England Hospital for Women and Children, first African-American trained nurse
1893	The first Nurses' Settlement House founded in New York City by Lillian Wald and Mary Brewster
1899	Teachers College, Columbia University offers first post-graduate course for nurses
1900	The *American Journal of Nursing* begins publication
1901	Army Nurse Corps created
1903	North Carolina passes first state nurse registration law
1904	The *Pacific Coast Journal of Nursing* begins publication
1908	Associate Alumnae defeats organizational support of suffrage resolution at eleventh annual convention in San Francisco
1908	Navy Nurse Corps created
1909	American Federation of Nurses defeats an organizational support for suffrage
1909	*Public Health Nurses Quarterly* begins publication
1910	Isabel Hamptom Robb dies in an accident, April 15
1911	University of Minnesota offers first collegiate program for basic nursing education
1912	The Associated Alumnae vote at the fifteenth annual convention to support suffrage at the next ICN conference
1912	Town and Country Rural Nursing Service created
1915	National League of Nursing Education (NLNE) and the American Nurses' Association (ANA) pass suffrage resolutions in support of the Susan B. Anthony bill in Congress
1918	NLNE executive board meeting passes resolution sanctioning the federal suffrage amendment on May 11
1920	The Federal Suffrage Amendment passes in Congress, August

Appendix H

Timeline:
Professional Nursing Organizations

1888	Alumnae association formed at the Training School of the Woman's Hospital in Philadelphia
1889	Alumnae association formed at the Training School for Nurses attached to Bellevue Hospital, New York
1891	Alumnae association formed at Illinois Training School
1892	Alumnae association formed at Johns Hopkins Training School
1893	American Society of Superintendents of Training Schools for Nurses (Superintendents' Society) formed
1893	Farrand Training School Alumnae Association formed at Harper Hospital in Detroit
1893	Congress of Hospitals and Dispensaries meet at the World's Columbian Exposition; Isabel Hampton Robb chairs nursing section
1895	Alumnae association formed at Massachusetts General Hospital nurse training school
	Alumnae Association of the Training School for Nurses of the Long Island College Hospital formed
1896	Nurses' Associated Alumnae of United States and Canada (Associated Alumnae)
1896	Alumnae association formed at Boston City Hospital nurse training school
1899	International Council of Nurses formed
1908	National Association of Colored Graduate Nurses (NACGN) formed
1911	Associated Alumnae renamed the American Nurses' Association (ANA)
1912	Superintendents' Society renamed the National League of Nursing Education (NLNE)

1912   National Organization for Public Health Nursing (NOPHN) formed
1951   NACGN dissolves and joins the ANA
1952   The National League of Nursing Education combines with the Association of Collegiate Schools of Nursing, the National Organization for Public Health Nursing, and National League for Nursing

Appendix I

Timeline:
Opening of Nurses Training Schools

1863   Charter granted to the New England Hospital for Women, Boston, Massachusetts

1871   New York State Training School for Nurses, Brooklyn Maternity, Brooklyn, NY

1872   New England Hospital for Women offers a one-year training program for nurses; Linda Richards becomes "America's first trained nurse"

1873   Opening of first Nightingale-influenced training schools:

— the New York Training School (later known as the Bellevue Training School) at Bellevue Hospital, New York

— the Connecticut Training School for Nurses at New Haven, CT

— the Boston Training School for Nurses at Massachusetts General Hospital

— Prospect Heights Hospital in Brooklyn

1875   Charity Hospital, New York City; Pennsylvania Hospital, Philadelphia

1877   New York Hospital, New York City

Hartford Hospital, Hartford, CT

Boston City Hospital, Boston

Buffalo General Hospital, Buffalo, NY

1878   Brooklyn Homeopathic Hospital, Brooklyn, NY

1880   Rochester City Hospital, Rochester, NY

Brooklyn Hospital, Brooklyn, NY

1882   Mary Fletcher Hospital, Burlington, VT

Orange Memorial Hospital, Orange, NJ

1883	Long Island College Hospital, Brooklyn, NY
	Cincinnati Training-School, Cincinnati, OH
	Charleston City Hospital, Charleston, SC
	Johns Hopkins Hospital, Baltimore, MD
	Farrand Training School for Nurses, Harper Hospital, Detroit, MI
1886	Spelman Seminary, Atlanta, GA
1888	Mills Training School for Men attached to Bellevue Hospital, New York
	Methodist Episcopal Hospital in Brooklyn
1891	Provident Hospital, Chicago
	Hampton Institute, Hampton, VA
1895	Frederick Douglass Memorial Hospital and Training School
1897	Kings County Hospital in Brooklyn, NY
1900	German Hospital (Wyckoff Heights Hospital) in Brooklyn, NY
1906	Brooklyn Jewish Hospital, Brooklyn, NY
1907	Mercy Hospital School for Nurses, Philadelphia
	Washington Training School, Washington, DC

Illustrations

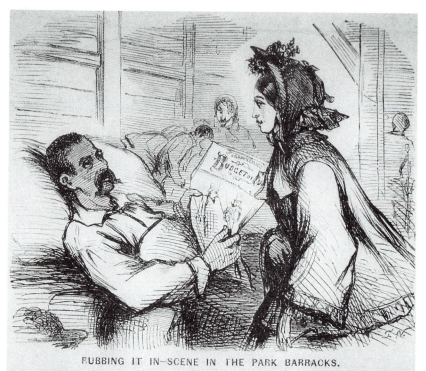

RUBBING IT IN—SCENE IN THE PARK BARRACKS.

Dramatis Personæ—A sick and wounded, but good-looking soldier, and an anxious lady nurse in search of a subject:

LADY NURSE—*" My poor fellow, can I do anything for you?"*

SOLDIER—(emphatically)—*" No, ma'am! Nothin'!"*

LADY NURSE—*" I should like to do something for you. Shall I not sponge your face and brow for you?"*

SOLDIER (despairingly)—*" You may if you want to very bad; but you'll be the fourteenth lady as has done it this blessed mornin'."*

Rubbing it in—scene in the park barracks. From Frank Leslie's *Illustrated Newspaper*—June 21, 1862.

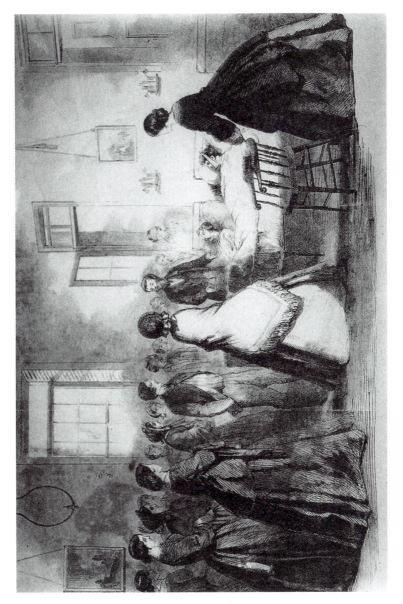

The Volunteer Nurses visiting the New York City Hospital, preparatory to joining the Hospital Department of the National Army. Undated and unnamed newspaper clipping—Lewenson Collection.

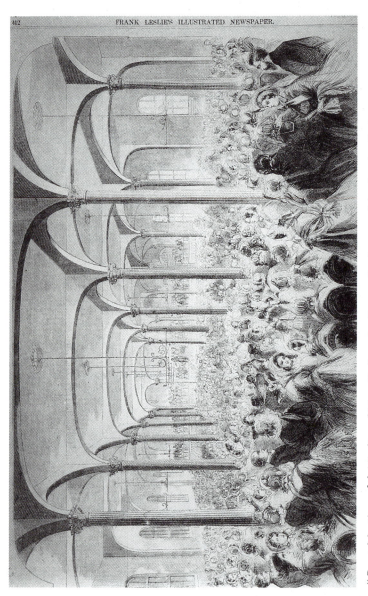

"Great Meeting of the Ladies of New York at the Cooper Institute on Monday April 29, 1861. To organize a society to be called 'Woman's Central Association of Relief.' To make clothes, lint, bandages, and to furnish nurses for the soldiers of the Northern Army." From Frank Leslie's Illustrated Newspaper, undated—Lewenson collection.

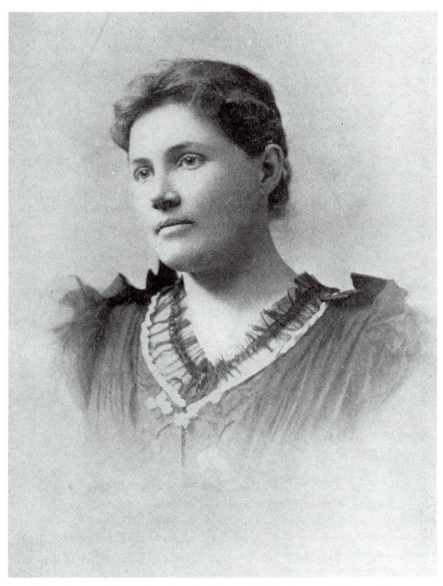

Isabel A. Hampton. From the *American Journal of Nursing,* vol. 11, no. 1 (October, 1910): 78–79. Courtesy of the *American Journal of Nursing.*

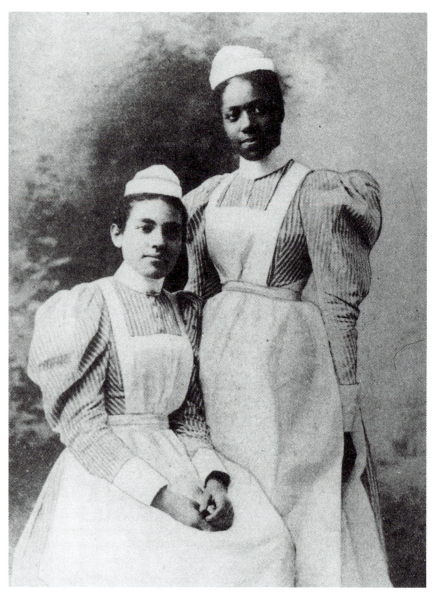

First graduate nurses from the Frederick Douglas Memorial Hospital and Training School, Philadelphia, 1897. Courtesy of the Center for the Study of the History of Nursing, University of Pennsylvania.

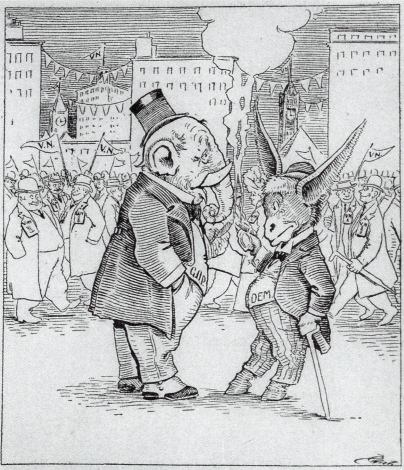

Loaned by *The Survey*.

G. O. P. to Dem.—I don't know who this *V. N.* is, but she's getting all the votes to-day.—*Minneapolis Journal.*
"*V. N.*" was the visiting nurse fund of the Minneapolis Associated Charities which raised money by a successful tag day.—*The Survey.*

Suffrage cartoon loaned by The Survey. From the *American Journal of Nursing,* vol. 11, no. 4 (January, 1911): 290–291. Courtesy of the *American Journal of Nursing.*

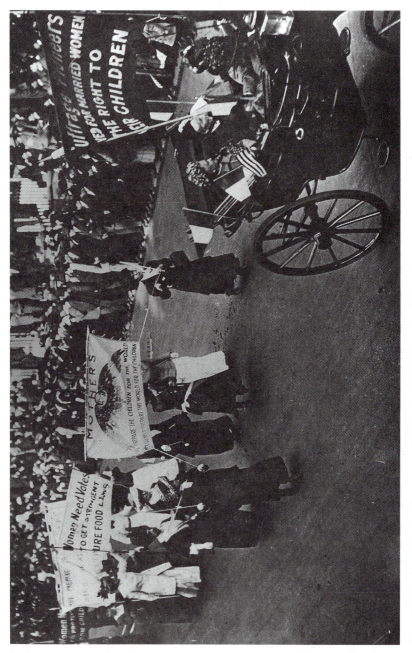

New York Suffrage Parade. Courtesy of the New York Historical Society.

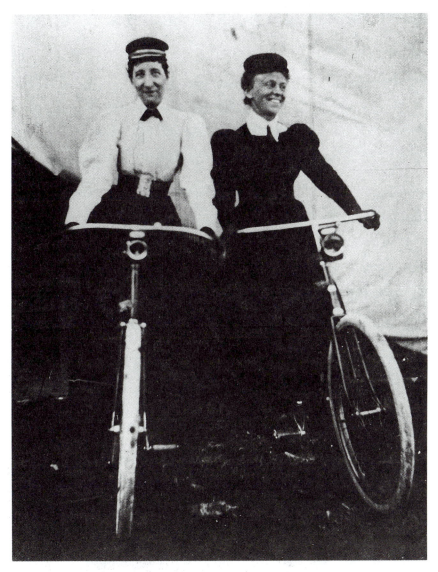

Lavinia Dock and Miss Fay, 1893 in Chicago. Courtesy of Special Collections, Milbank Memorial Library, Teachers College, Columbia University.

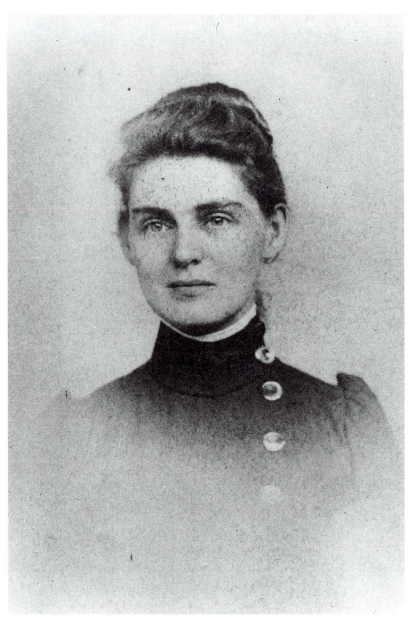

Mary Adelaide Nutting in a Johns Hopkins Hack uniform. Courtesy of Special Collections, Milbank Memorial Library, Teachers College, Columbia University.

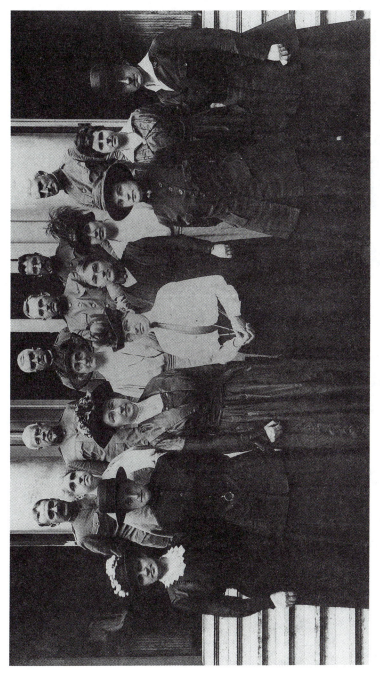

Council of National Defense, General Medical Board, Committee on Nursing, WWI, 1918; includes Annie Goodrich, Mary Beard, Jane Delano, and Mary Adelaide Nutting. Courtesy of Special Collections, Milbank Memorial Library, Teachers College, Columbia University.

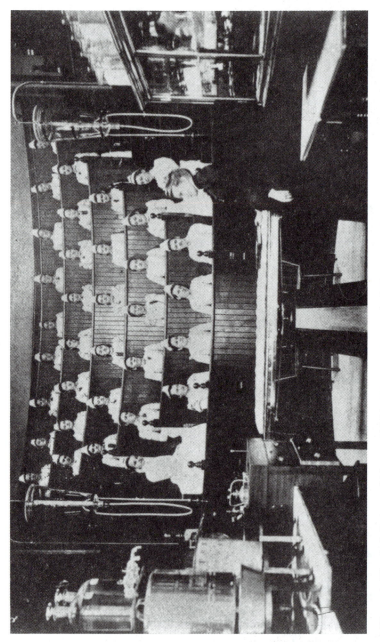

Woman's Hospital clinic amphitheatre, 1892. Woman's Hospital of Philadelphia Records. Courtesy of the Center for the Study of the History of Nursing, University of Pennsylvania.

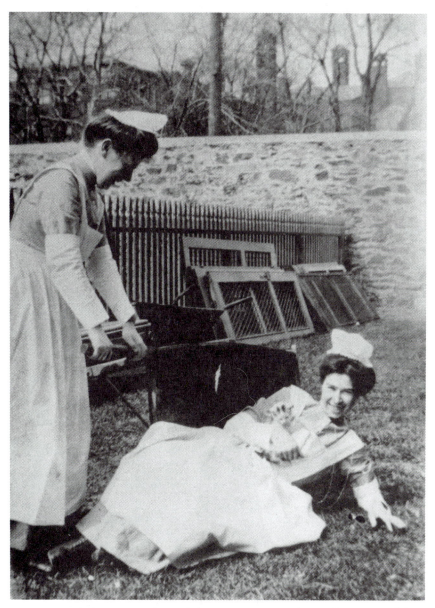

Two unidentified nurses at play with kitten, ca. 1910. Alumni Association of the Training School for Nurses of Philadelphia General Hospital Collection. Courtesy of the Center for the Study of the History of Nursing, University of Pennsylvania.

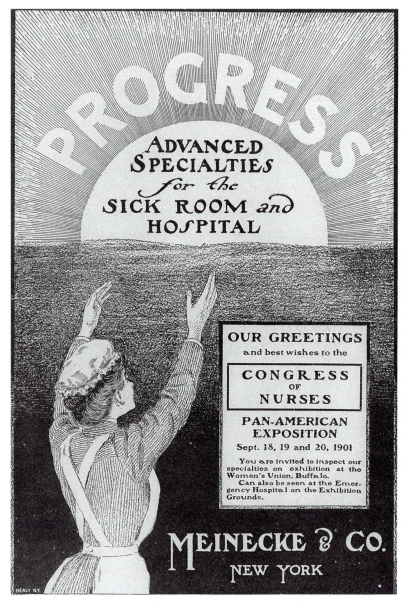

The advertisement—"Progress" with special greetings to the Nurses Congress (at the ICN first meeting in Buffalo, New York). From the *American Journal of Nursing,* vol. 1, no. 12 (September 1901). Courtesy of the *American Journal of Nursing.*

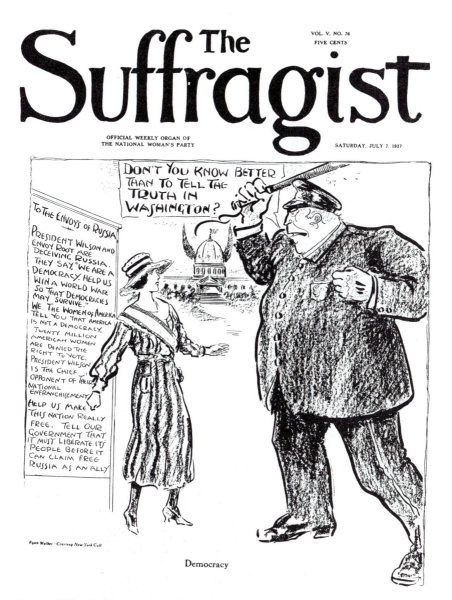

Cover of The Suffragist. *Saturday, July 7, 1917.* Courtesy of Social Welfare History Archives, University Libraries, University of Minnesota.

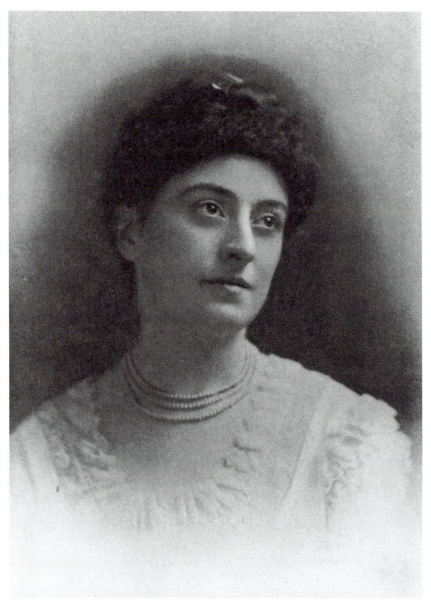

Ethel Gordon Fenwick, President International Council of Nurses and Honorary President of Congress. From the *American Journal of Nursing,* vol. 1, no. 12, September 1901, opp. page 861. Courtesy of the *American Journal of Nursing.*

Index

Index

Other Books of Interest from NLN Press

You may order NLN books by • TELEPHONE 800-NOW-9NLN, ext. 138
• Fax 212-989-3710 • MAIL Simply use the order form below

Book Title	Pub. No.	Price	NLN Member Price
☐ **The Path We Tread: Blacks in Nursing Worldwide, 1854–1994** *by M. Elizabeth Carnegie*	14-2678	$30.95	$27.95
☐ **African American Voices** *Edited by Ruth Johnson*	14-2631	32.95	29.95
☐ **Hispanic Voices** *Edited by Sara Torres*	14-2693	32.95	29.95
☐ **The Emergence of Women into the 21st Century** *Edited by Patricia L. Munhall & Virginia M. Fitzsimons*	14-6622	25.95	23.95
☐ **Peace and Power: Building Communities for the Future** *by Peggy L. Chinn*	14-2697	16.95	14.95
☐ **Legacy of Leadership** *Edited by Nettie Birnback & Sandra Lewenson*	14-2514	39.95	35.95

PHOTOCOPY THIS FORM TO ORDER BY MAIL OR FAX

Photocopy this coupon and send with 1) a check payable to NLN, 2) credit card information, or 3) a purchase order number to: **NLN Publications Order Unit, 350 Hudson Street, New York, NY 10014 (FAX: 212-989-3710).**

Shipping & Handling via UPS Ground				
Amount	Charges	Amount	Charges
Up to $10.99	$ 2.65	75.00–99.99	8.15
11.00–24.99	3.95	100.00–124.99	9.45
25.00–49.99	5.50	125.00–149.99	11.05
50.00–74.99	6.85	250.00 and up	15.75

Subtotal: $ _____

Shipping & Handling
(see chart): $ _____

Total: $ _____

☐ Check enclosed   ☐ P.O. # _____   NLN Member # (if appl.): _____

Charge the above total to   ☐ Visa   ☐ MasterCard   ☐ American Express

Acct. #: _____   Exp. Date: _____

Authorized Signature: _____

Name _____   Title _____

Institution _____

Address _____

City, State, Zip _____

Daytime Telephone (____) _____   Ext. _____